THE ROLE OF
CHIROPRACTIC

Leonard W. Rutherford, D.C.

Published by Health Education Publishing Corp., Box 2388, Eugene, Oregon 97402

Printed by
The Clinton Press Inc.
500 West 12th Street
Erie, Pennsylvania 16501

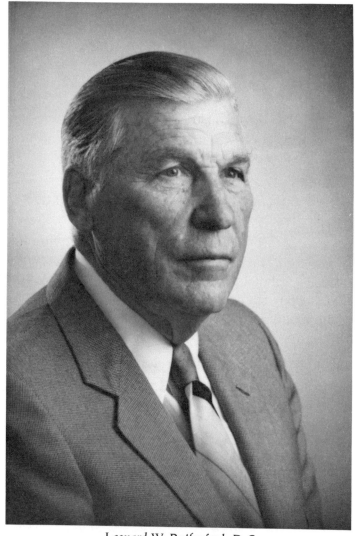

Leonard W. Rutherford, D.C.

During the preceding years, I have been active in the profession and have made major contributions in the establishment and excellence of the profession of chiropractic.

I enrolled as a student in the Palmer School of Chiropractic in 1936.

Following my graduation, I practiced in Eugene, Oregon, retiring after 31 years of active practice.

While in practice, I was involved in many professional activities. I was a member of the Representatives Assembly from the State of Oregon for the Chiropractic Health Bureau and its successor organization, the International Chiropractors Association, 1941-1951.

In 1951, I was elected to the Board of Control of the International Chiropractors Association, carrying on in this capacity for the following ten years, until 1961.

In 1961-1964, I was elected Vice President of the International Chiropractors Association.

In 1964, I was elected President of the International Chiropractors Association. In all, I was elected to three consecutive terms as President of the Association, 1964-1971.

Only Dr. B. J. Palmer, served the organization as president for a longer period of time than myself.

Following my years as president of the Association, I moved to Chairman of the Board of the Association from 1971-1975. I received many honors over the years. To name a few:

    A. Fellow of the International Chiropractors Association.

    B. The prestigious award, Chiropractor of the Year, given by the Association.

    C. The Doctor of Chiropractic Humanities (HCD).

I served as a member of the Board of Trustees of Palmer College of Chiropractic from the inception of the Board until my resignation in 1978.

Early in my chiropractic career, I was introduced to and witnessed blatant, unqualified invasion of medical and physical therapy practices by those whose only desire was to be a chiropractic physician.

Over a three year period of time, six months of which was spent interning in the B. J. Palmer Research Clinic, Davenport, Iowa, I learned the philosophy, science and art of chiropractic. I received my diploma from the Palmer School of Chiropractic with D. C. (Doctor of Chiropractic degree).

I then enrolled in Western States College and received a diploma for post graduate courses in Electrotherapy, Hydrotherapy and Physiotherapy.

This schooling would fulfill the requirements of the Oregon Statutes relative to chiropractic and make me proficient in the eyes of the Board of Examiners to practice the following: physical therapy, including electrotherapy, hydrotherapy, diathermy, short wave therapy, ultra sound therapy, minor surgery, tonsil coagulation, eye, ear, nose and throat practice, colon irrigation, hemorrhoidal treatment, a foot and ankle exercising practice, all of these and other similar related practices.

What a farce! But further, what a potential danger to public health awaited the unsuspecting public who sought such services. The training I received qualified me for none of these practices, even if I had wanted to do them, which I did not in any manner.

I purchased one book, Electro-therapy and Light Therapy by Kovacs. A card table was my desk. I was the only student taking the 'course' at that time. I never did know who was supposed to be the instructor.

However, the education I received in the practices qualified me to write the State Board Examinations. I was successful in doing so. I received my license to practice chiropractic in the State of Oregon. Having received one of the highest grades of any who at that time took the examination, I was awarded a picture from the Board of Examiners with the inscription, "The Dawn of Hope". The painting expresses the gratitude of a lady who recovered her health through chiropractic after all other healing methods had failed.

My chiropractic license was signed by John E. LaValley, D.C. along with the other members of the Board of Examiners.

John E. LaValley, D.C. was an associate of D. D. Palmer when D. D. Palmer founded his school of Chiropractic in Portland, Oregon. He was a strong supporter and advocate of the philosophy and principles of chiropractic as propounded by D. D. Palmer.

My friendship with Dr. LaValley gave me a very unique, special understanding of D. D. Palmer, the Founder of our profession. I felt that I could almost go back to the beginning of chiropractic - 1895 and 1939 didn't seem so far apart. And D. D. Palmer had passed away only in 1913.

I am proud to say that over the many years which I was privileged to take care of thousands of patients, my practice was confined strictly to chiropractic.

The three months of pseudo-training, seeing first

hand the molding of the "MIXER" chiropractic physician, crystallized my determination to use my efforts to help the true role of chiropractic. For indeed, chiropractic confined within its own principles and practice has a tremendous potential for service in the healing professions.

So it was that the conflicting intra struggle within the profession was brought 'up front' to me very early in my chiropractic career.

I was at that time, and still remain firmly committed to the protection and preservation of chiropractic within the true intent of its principles and practice.

As has been said many times, 'nothing is so powerful as an idea whose time has come.' In my life, chiropractic's time had come, and the time had come for chiropractic.

I resolved then and there that my time and talents would be utilized in keeping and projecting chiropractic as a separate practice. In this manner a freedom of choice in the healing arts might be maintained for those in need of health services. Chiropractic would have the opportunity to prove its worth in service to humanity.

For chiropractic adds years to life and life to years—I am living proof of these words.

To my wife, Agnes, my helpmate and companion through the years; To our children, William, Mary, Gayle and Alan who "understood" when Dad was gone on his many travels for chiropractic;

To my grandchildren, some of whom may pursue chiropractic as a career;

To the pioneers of yesterday, who stood for chiropractic, many willing to go to jail for the right to practice—you, who are gone but not forgotten:

To the pioneers of today—chiropractors carrying the "singleness of purpose" of the chiropactic profession;

To the millions of people who have and will benefit from spinal adjustments and who have spread the message of help in health matters from this great profession;

To you who have helped in the preparation of this work;

And to you of tomorrow, who will again chart a new course in keeping a freedom of choice in the healing professions.

To you, this work is dedicated—May it serve a purpose.

FORWARD

Dr. Leonard W. Rutherford has been an able and effective spokesman for Chiropractic, and particularly so during the early formative years of the Federal Employee Health Benefits Program. He has always had a highly developed ability to educate the uninformed, and to present and defend a point of view.

Now, his book, *"The Role of Chiropractic"* will continue the educational mission he began over twenty-five years ago. It should prove most helpful to his peers in the profession, as well as to insurance administrators and planners who are interested in maximum utilization of scarce premium dollars.

Andrew E. Ruddock
Former Director, Bureau of Retirement,
Insurance, and Occupational Health
United States Civil Service Commission

Dr. Rutherford's work on chiropractic will mark a watershed in the history of the chiropractic profession. ''*The Role of Chiropractic*'' delineates the direction which the profession must take to gain public-wide acceptance and full governmental recognition, not only as a weapon in man's arsenal against pain and disease but also as a full partner with the traditional modalities of medical practice in securing to all people the benefits of improved health care to which they are entitled.

''*The Role of Chiropractic*'' illuminates the path not only for the profession but for those in government and in the insurance industry as well, so all may see that it is only through the disciplined character of true chiropractic that the vast potential of this science to help mankind can be realized.

Irving Kator
Senior Member, Kator, Scott & Heller, Chtd.
Former Assistant Executive Director,
U.S. Civil Service Commission

CONTENTS

CHAPTER I

INTRODUCTION

My somersault from the beam in the barn to the pile of hay below was not fulfilled. I missed the body roll necessary to land on my feet. My knee struck my eye, forcing my head back violently. Every bone in my neck seemed to break with a loud cracking noise.

At first I thought I had, in fact, broken my neck. However, after help from my friends in getting up and after being able to turn my head from side to side, we decided that this had not happened. My eye and the area around it was beginning to discolor and blacken. My neck stiffened. Turning my head was painful and difficult. These symptoms would persist for many weeks.

The year was 1929, and I was a teenager growing up on a farm in the Hazel Green District near Salem, Oregon.

My condition soon worsened. Shortly after the accident, I developed heart trouble. I became very worried. Never before in my fifteen years had I experienced any kind of a health problem. Growing up on our farm, I had been able to help my family with the work in any manner needed. The fall in the loft of our neighbor's barn had not just demonstrated my shortcomings as a gymnast; it had caused a serious health crisis. Severe pains and irregular rhythm began and persisted in my heart.

Night time was the worst of times. Night after night, I would lay in bed trying to sleep. I would listen to the irregular thumping of my heart and try to endure the pain.

I even lost weight. Finally, I was literally skin and bones, and I was constantly nervous. School was out of the question. I had to drop out of my high school classes. My condition was becoming critical. There was no question in my mind or in the mind of my parents that if something were not done to help me, I would not live long.

Our family medical doctor checked me and prescribed medicine. We also consulted other specialists who prescribed other medicines. It became obvious that something more had to be done if I were to live and regain my health.

Finally and luckily, my parents took me to a chiropractor. His name was Dr. O. L. Scott, and his offices were in Salem, Oregon. Dr. Scott was a large, robust man who had absolute confidence in the healing powers of chiropractic. His procedure was entirely different from our family medical doctor.

Instead of checking my pulse, listening to my heart, or taking my blood pressure; Dr. Scott examined my spine, particularly the back of my neck. This area was still very sore and tender. In his examination, he used an instrument which he glided up my spine. Later I would learn that this instrument was called a neurocalometer. It registered a large temperature differential reading on the sides of my spine and in my upper neck region. The closer he came to the back of my head, the more painful and tender it felt. Then he took X-ray pictures of my neck area.

The following day we returned to his office. Dr. Scott told my folks that my neck bones were so badly out of position that at first he thought I had completely dislocated the atlas (uppermost vertebra). "You can give this boy all the medicine in the world, and it will not correct the problem," he told my folks. He said he found the first and second cervical vertebrae (those right at the top of my neck and under my skull) to be severely out of place. In chiropractic, this is called a 'subluxation'. (A subluxation means a vertebra out of proper alignment causing a pressure or an interference on the nervous system). My fall had forced the first vertebra out of its normal position in the articulations that connected it to the occipital bone of the skull. The second vertebra had also been shifted out of its normal position. The X-ray plates revealed a severe misalignment of these bones in my neck.

But there were still other problems. Dr. Scott explained further that the out-of-place bones of my spine were causing a pressure and disturbance on my nervous system. The neurocalometer also indicated a heat differential in the second and third dorsal region of my spine. It was Dr. Scott's feeling, however, that the severe misalignment of my upper neck was the primary factor causing my trouble. The bones which were out of place in my upper neck were pressuring the nerves supplying my heart region. This pressure had caused my heart trouble.

After explaining the problem he had found, Dr. Scott placed me on his adjusting table. Using only his hands, he adjusted my neck bones. After this adjustment, he placed me under his care for the necessary checkups and further adjustments.

In a short while, I began to feel better. My heart trouble cleared up. My appetite returned. I gained weight and began to feel like myself again. I enrolled in high school. Before long I was well. Life was once again worth living.

This experience was my personal introduction to the profession of chiropractic. I have no doubt that chiropractic saved my life. I was cured completely, and I took no drugs or medicines. All the chiropractor did was adjust my neck bones. When he had properly adjusted these spinal bones, the pressure was released from the pinched nerves. My heart trouble cleared up completely.

My somersault accident brought me in touch with a mode of healing which was later to be my life's work.

I would never forget this experience. During my forty-eight years of involvement in the chiropractic profession, I witnessed innumerable occasions where chiropractic produced tremendous results in health restoration. The thousands of patients whom I aided with chiropractic proved to me and to them that spinal adjustments play a key role in solving many health problems.

But whenever I think of the past, I am saddened by the deplorable state-of-affairs in which chiropractic finds itself today.

There is absolutely no doubt in my mind that chiropractic is extremely beneficial to human health. The history of chiropractic testifies to that fact. Nevertheless, virtually the entire history of chiropractic has been burdened by disrespect from other healing professions, public suspicion, judicial and legislative challenges and, sometimes, charges of "quackery". Most of this disrespect and most of these charges are absolutely unjustified.

But some ARE justified.

THE ROLE OF CHIROPRACTIC tells why. This book

examines the history of chiropractic, both past and recent. It shows where chiropractic has earned praise and respect, but it also shows where it has earned criticism and it shows why.

Throughout all strata of our society, a great deal of confusion exists about the proper role of chiropractic. This book seeks to end that confusion. This book seeks to give definition and direction to the chiropractic profession. It attempts to lead chiropractic toward the public respect and confidence it deserves.

There has never been any question in my mind but that chiropractic has a right to be included among the services provided by the healing professions. Still, I have never had a parochial attitude about chiropractic; I have never come to the conclusion that chiropractic alone can solve every health problem. I never attempted to perform services for which I had not been trained. Any individual who did not need chiropractic care was always so advised.

But, I am sad to acknowledge that today there are many chiropractic licentiates who are, in fact, quite willing to engage in services for which they have no real training or accreditation. Whether they intend it or not, these individuals are the major cause of the public disrespect to the chiropractic profession.

Therefore, one of the major themes of this book is that the "mixing" of chiropractic with medical therapies, with physical therapies, and with other practices foreign to chiropractic is one of the major causes of the chiropractic profession's problems. Briefly defined, 'mixing' is the combining of chiropractic services with other professional practices which cannot in any way be construed as chiropractic; practices which a chiropractor is neither trained nor qualified to perform. I believe mixing is the source of much of chiropractic's justified disrespect, and the source of many of its justified charges of "quackery."

If every member of the chiropractic profession would confine practice within the legitimate chiropractic field of practice, the confusion about the proper role of chiropractic would not exist as it does today.

Throughout the world, patients seeking chiropractic care can only be left in a most confused state of mind when they confront the many different modes of chiropractic care.

In some states, chiropractic practice is confined to the true role of chiropractic, spinal analysis and spinal adjusting.

But in other states, chiropractors and chiropractic physicians practice minor surgery, obstetrics, physiotherapy, electrotherapy, hydrotherapy, massage, dietetics, casting of fractures, colonic irrigation, disc treatment, nutritional remedies, wholistic health care, acupuncture, hemorrhoidal treatment, vitamin therapy, and a host of other practices foreign to chiropractic.

When mixers attempt to perform these services, it becomes a shameful mockery to chiropractic. And what a shame that it is all unnecessary and unjustified!

Unfortunately, the impetus for mixing does not just come from unscrupulous chiropractors. Respected institutions also assist the proliferation of mixing.

In legal decisions, courts have defined chiropractic as separate and distinct from other practices. But this is not always the case in legislative decisions. In my opinion, no other profession is allowed such a latitude of practices by the various legislative bodies. And no other profession is so poorly qualified in meeting accredited educational standards for non-chiropractic practices as is the chiropractic profession. Under many legislative statutes, chiropractors are allowed to practice various medical and physical therapy practices foreign to chiropractic and giving the public the false impression that they possess adequate accreditation in those practices, when, in fact, they do not. Surely, those who seek the services chiropractic has to offer should be assured that the chiropractor stays within the bounds of proper professional practice. The public not only deserves but should demand these qualifcations and protection.

But a primary reason mixing goes on in the chiropractic profession is because mixing is being taught in chiropractic colleges. Some chiropractic colleges are teaching physical therapy, electrotherapy, hydrotherapy, colonic irrigation, casting of fractures, proctology, minor surgery, gynecology, nutrition, obstetrics, pediatrics, and otolaryngology. In some of these colleges, laboratory practices include: phlebotomy, EKG, glucose tolerance test, and hematology.

I strongly believe that chiropractic colleges should confine their teaching to the principles and practice inherent within chiropractic's separate and distinct profession. Chiropractic colleges should teach chiropractic rather than attempting to involve the student in other professional practices that fail to meet the accreditation standards for those practices.

Today, chiropractic stands at a crossroad. A flaming controversy exists within the profession sparked by the ongoing conflict between the straight and mixer factions within the profession. The vital questions are these: Will chiropractic confine itself to its own principles and practices embodied in spinal analysis and spinal adjustments (as propounded by the straight segment of the profession)? Or will chiropractic continue its attempts to invade and usurp the practices of other professions (as propounded by the mixer segment of the profession)?

I have been in the chiropractic profession for almost half a century. This book presents the knowledge I have acquired during that time. During these years, I served in many capacities within the profession, including six years as President of the International Chiropractors Association. I worked closely with Dr. B. J. Palmer, the Developer of chiropractic. Dr. David D. Palmer, the Chiropractic Educator and grandson of the Founder of Chiropractic was also a close associate. He and I were members of the same graduating class at Palmer College of Chiropractic. I have worked with government programs, with the legal profession, with insurance programs, and with education to help establish chiropractic in its rightful role.

It will be obvious in this book that I have strong opinions about the proper role of the chiropractor. I am a "straight" chiropractor, and I am proud to affirm that fact. Still, THE ROLE OF CHIROPRACTIC attempts to provide an objective view of the chiropractic profession. It poses questions: What is the limitation of chiropractic? What is the role of chiropractic in the health professions?

In the following pages, I present a panoramic view of the chiropractic profession:

• I present a concise overview of the current controversy in the chiropractic profession involving the "mixer" chiropractic versus the "straight" chiropractic. I discuss how the mixing segment of the chiropractic profession attempts to include the practices of other professions under the banner of chiropractic.

- I describe the history of chiropractic from its humble beginning in 1895, to its vast areas of recognition and acceptance today. This history surveys chiropractic's struggle to attain its place in the healing arts as a separate, distinct school of healing. I share the words of the Founder of Chiropractic, D. D. Palmer as he writes of his discoveries. In this book, I quote Dr. B. J. Palmer and his voluminous writings on the development of chiropractic. I describe Dr. David D. Palmer's vital contributions to chiropractic education.

- In a chapter on Chiropractic and the Law, I present ample evidence that, legally, chiropractic is a separate and distinct practice. I show the need for legislative statutes that clarify and identify the proper role of the profession.

- For the lay reader's understanding, I provide a description of chiropractic by describing a typical visit to a chiropractor's office. I demonstrate the healing potential of spinal adjustment by describing successful case histories I personally experienced in my practice.

- I describe the current status of chiropractic education and how the "mixer" philosophy has suffused that education. I probe the tremendous controversy over chiropractic accreditation as it affects both educational institutions and aspiring chiropractors.

- I show how the profession should "police" itself to avoid charges of "quackery".

- In a chapter on insurance, I again stress the importance of keeping chiropractic within its proper scope of practice. I describe my many years of work which resulted in chiropractic being accepted by the U.S. Civil Service Commission, as well as by many labor unions and insurance companies. The inclusion of chiropractic services in Medicare was also a top priority program. These were years when I attempted to inform the insurance industry about the merits of chiropractic.

- In concluding chapters, I attempt to envision a future path for chiropractic; how chiropractic can achieve a respected professional status, and what I see as the future accomplishments of chiropractic research.

- It is my hope that this book will give readers a complete understanding of the chiropractic profession. The path I have traveled in my career has led me through many experiences. Many lives have touched mine and influenced my career. I, in turn, have been privileged to touch many lives and hopefully to influence the future role of chiropractic.

CHAPTER II

UNDERSTANDING CHIROPRACTIC

GOD GAVE US HANDS

God gave us hands
To hold, and heal
To touch, and work
And play.

The hands He gave
Are the links between,
Each child, and woman, and man
As we travel the road
He laid for us
To fulfill the master plan.

L. W. Rutherford

The little girl was blind. It was a tremendously unfair burden and tragedy for a five-year old to endure. She was attending a school for the blind, learning as best she could to cope with all obstacles life might hold. Her parents were desperate. Everything and every type of healing had been tried but to no avail. Their child seemed doomed to a life of perpetual darkness.

When the little girl's parents brought her to me, I had opened my chiropractic office in Eugene, Oregon, in 1939, and had been in practice less than two years. The knowledge I had gained during my internship in the B. J. Palmer Chiropractic Research Clinic was proving most valuable in helping patients who came to me.

Somehow, somewhere, the parents of this little girl had heard of me and of what I had done for others. They called for an appointment.

I shall never forget meeting this sweet little brownhaired girl who was unable to see. She truly touched me personally.

After checking her spine with instruments, I located an interference in the neck region, close to the skull. I then x-rayed the area. Soon I verified that, indeed, there was a subluxation. The top most vertebra was out of normal position. This was causing an interference on the nervous system at that level of the spine.

I explained my findings to the parents. We agreed that I would try to adjust the subluxated vertebra. It might be the answer to their little girl's loss of sight.

I made the adjustment. I adjusted her only one time and in one place. That was all.

Amazingly, I then saw what seemed like a miracle: her sight returned. I will never forget that moment nor would the parents and the child. It was indeed a miracle. When her sight returned, the little girl cried out to her mother and father: "I can see you. Really I can. Now I know what you look like."

They all cried together. It was a touching moment. As mother and father held her close, they handled her like a china doll, lest something should happen to again rob her of her precious sight. From that day on, her eyesight continued to be good.

Apparently, news of my restoration of the little girl's sight spread. Eventually, it would cause me to receive a deferment during World War II.

One day, I received a phone call. It was an invitation

to the home of Oregon's late Senior Senator, Charles L. McNary. He knew the parents of the blind little girl I had helped, and he wanted to talk to me.

When I met the Senator, we talked for some time. Finally, he asked me what would happen if I were inducted into the military service. I explained to him that chiropractic was not recognized by the military. I would probably be assigned as an x-ray technician or something similar.

After listening, he said: "Your work is too valuable to lose." He told me he would do whatever he could to help me keep in practice so that I could go on helping people.

Senator McNary then contacted General George Hershey in Washington, D.C. Hershey made other contacts and, eventually, arranged for me to receive an "essential service" deferment from President Franklin D. Roosevelt.

My deferment was the first in my profession, and it led the way for others.

All of this happened because of a spinal adjustment that restored sight to the little five-year old girl.

Some time ago, I received a letter from the girl whom I had helped. The letter read:

> Dear Dr. Rutherford:
> Today is my birthday which may be my reason for feeling so grateful for my eyesight and my life, and grateful to you who gave me my good health. I will be forever grateful to you.
> Today is such a lovely day.

Chiropractors understand that the body has an innate power to heal itself. Who knows the capacity of the innate power within each of us in its role of healing?

The memories of the many patients who have come to me have left an indelible impression in my mind. I share some of these memories with you, the reader, so that you might better understand the full importance and the full potential of chiropractic.

I would be less than candid if I told you that I helped everyone who came to me. But, always, if it seemed that the patient needed other types of professional help, I referred the patient to someone in the appropriate field. Any individual who did not need chiropractic care was always so advised.

When I found interference due to subluxated vertebrae, and when I determined that I could safely and accurately adjust the subluxation, I did so. The innate power within the body was released to accomplish healing and health restoration.

In the subsequent chapters, it will become obvious that I am very critical of what is often defined as "chiropractic." Nevertheless, if I am going to criticize what I feel improper in chiropractic, I must give the reader a complete understanding of what in my opinion constitutes proper chiropractic.

To aid this understanding, let me describe a typical visit to a chiropractor's office. As an example, suppose you are visiting the office of John Doe, D.C. (Doctor of Chiropractic). Dr. Doe is a straight chiropractor and practices chiropractic within the confines of the principles and practices as established by the Palmers.

Perhaps, you have decided to consult a chiropractor because other methods and healing professions have failed to answer your health problems. Perhaps, you have heard of the work done by chiropractors, and you came either on recommendation or because you feel chiropractic can solve your particular health problem.

Dr. Doe is, indeed, a straight chiropractor. Do not expect him to use medical procedures, physical therapy procedures, or any other professional practices as a part of his chiropractic service.

You explain to Dr. Doe that you have a problem. For the purposes of this example, let us say you have been diagnosed medically as having stomach trouble—gastritis or ulcers.

How could chiropractic help stomach trouble?

Dr. Doe explains to you that every organ and tissue of the body is controlled by the brain through the nervous system. To ascertain whether or not vertebrae may be out of their normal position, causing a nerve pressure or interference to nerves supplying the stomach, he explains that he will examine your spine. Chiropractic adds nothing to the body, nor does it take anything away. And through spinal adjustment, the chiropractor restores the vertebrae to normal position, this in turn releases pressures or interferences from the nervous system. The body then heals itself from within.

So how could your spine be involved when your stomach is part of your body that is giving you the pain and indigestion? Dr. Doe takes you over to a wall chart which illustrates the body, the spine, and the nerves.

Dr. Doe points out that the nervous system is an extension of the brain. As the spinal cord passes down the spine, it distributes nerves to all body parts. The stomach is innervated by nerves emitting from the 13th, 14th, 15th intervertebral foramina (mid-back region). He explains that impulses must be free to flow if the stomach and all body parts are to function normally. He compares this process to an electrical system with the brain as the power source or dynamo while the nerves are the wires. Electricity made by the dynamo flows over the wires and makes the motor, lights, etc. work.

If there is a short in the wires supplying the motor or a light, they fail to work. Essentially, the same thing can happen with your nervous system.

It is absolutely essential for there to be a normal energy flow over your nervous system if your stomach or any other part of your body is to function normally. You get the idea; a chiropractor is rather like an electrician for humans.

Once you understand how chiropractic works, you give Dr. Doe permission to see if he can be of help.

Dr. Doe has already heard your health history, noting your prior health treatments. He explains that drugs that kill pain, sleeping pills, etc. tend to affect the flow of energy over the nervous system, so he asks you about that. You inform him that you are not taking any medication.

Dr. Doe then proceeds with his analysis of the spine. To do this, he uses an instrument called a neurocalograph. This instrument is sensitive to minute amounts of heat. It records temperature differentials on the sides of the spine.

He begins his spinal checkup in the low back by gliding the instrument up the sides of the spine. The instrument is composed of a pickup unit with two poles (or pickups), one on each side of the spine. As the instrument glides up the spine, it makes a graph on a paper which flows from the recording section of the neurocalograph. Dr. Doe continues the gliding motion until he reaches the base of the skull. The resultant graph record is approximately 20 inches in length. He explains that in many instances a similar graph may be made on two or three separate office calls. This is to be certain that the graph pattern is consistent. He says this would be advisable in your case.

Two more visits confirm that the graph patterns are the same. The pattern is consistent. The instrument has located and graphed a large temperature differential in the lumbar area, in the mid-dorsal area, and in the upper cervical area of the spine. Dr. Doe explains that the uppermost area of temperature differential indicates an interruption to the impulse flow over the nervous system in the upper cervical spine. That, he says, is the primary interference. A pressure or interference at the higher level could well be the causation factor of the lower graph patterns. This makes sense to you because you remember the comparison Dr. Doe made with the dynamo. You ask if he is not going to do something to check your abdominal area, but he assures you that the medical care you have already received has completed those examinations. His work is to try to find the nerve interference which causes your problem.

Next, Dr. Doe takes you to the x-ray laboratory where he completes a series of x-ray plates of the upper cervical spine. Included in these x-rays are an anterior-posterior view, lateral view, stereoscopic diagonal, and base posterior views. Dr. Doe tells you to return another day when he will give you a report on his findings.

When you return, Dr. Doe explains the findings of his work. The neurocalograph located the interference at the first vertebral level (first or topmost vertebra). The x-rays revealed a severe misalignment of the atlas vertebra in relation to the occipital bone at the base of the skull and the axis or second vertebra. Dr. Doe explains that the misaligned vertebra is causing an interference on the spinal cord at that level. This, in turn, is causing the additional differential heat readings recorded on the graph. His analysis is an Atlas (first vertebra) subluxation.

Dr. Doe then places you on an adjusting chair (he mentions that some chiropractors use an adjusting table for the same purpose). As you are placed on the chair, there is little tension in your neck area, and you actually feel perfectly comfortable. But, of course, you are a bit anxious about what comes next.

Dr. Doe again studies the x-ray findings. He explains that with his hands he is going to make an adjustment (i.e., introduce the invasionary force in just the right amount and at the exact angles as ascertained by the x-ray plates. This will allow the muscles of your neck area to respond and to be utilized to establish the normal range-of-motion for the atlas vertebra). Dr. Doe then makes the adjustment. You find this adjustment is not uncomfortable. You may or may not hear a slight cracking noise as the vertebrae move. There is little or no pain or shock. In fact, you asked Dr. Doe: "Is that all you are going to do?"

He says, "Yes, for now!"

Dr. Doe explains that researchers in chiropractic have developed adjusting instruments to perform the spinal adjustment. At the present time, however, the vast majority of straight chiropractors ably employ the use of their hands in spinal adjusting.

Dr. Doe again re-checks you with the neurocalograph. He is very satisfied with your pattern of heat differential change following the adjustment. The nurse takes you to the dressing room where there is a comfortable bed. You lie on your back with a low pillow to keep all tensions off the neck muscles. You rest for about an hour.

Upon leaving the office, Dr. Doe explains that it usually takes about three weeks for the atlas area joints to heal and to regain normal muscle tone so that the vertebra will be held in its normal range. Dr. Doe gives you instructions not to lift heavy objects, to strain, or to do anything that might disturb the spine.

Further adjustments might be necessary, of course, if an interference develops on the nervous system. Dr. Doe places you under a program in which he will check you to be certain the vertebra will not again become subluxated.

As your nerve interference is released, you gradually begin to feel better. Soon your stomach symptoms subside and you have no stomach trouble. Internal healing has taken place.

This is a typical visit to a straight chiropractor.

But every chiropractor can tell you these stories, stories that reveal the tremendous versatility of chiropractic as a healing method. Most lay people associate spinal problems with back pain. But the fact is: spinal subluxations can cause many problems other than just back pain; problems, in fact, that would seem to be unrelated to spinal sublaxations.

Let me share some experiences from my own practice.

I recall a lady in her early twenties who came to see

me for help. She related a history of heart trouble: severe irregular beating or rhythm accompanied by pain in the area of the heart. Particularly, I recall what she told me regarding her difficulty in attempting to sleep. She said she felt that if she couldn't get up and out of bed several times during the night, she knew her heart would stop beating and she would die. Her heart irregularity and pain were very pronounced. Her family consisted of two young children and her husband. The husband was so distraught and disgusted with doctors that he did not come in at the time of the first conference. They had, as she told me, literally 'spent themselves poor on doctors'. None helped. As I listened to her story, I recalled my own heart problem many years before. Could I do the same for her as was done for me? I was certainly going to try.

In the spinal check-ups, instruments located the interference over the second and third dorsal or thoracic vertebrae. No other area of the spine indicated a problem. I x-rayed the area of the second and third dorsal vertebrae.

To my surprise, I found a large sewing needle, broken in several pieces and embedded deeply in the tissue of the spine. I could look right through the eye of that needle.

Upon returning for the report, the husband also came. I gave them the report showing them the x-ray plates with the needle embedded over the second and third vertebrae. I explained to them how the needle could be disturbing the nerve impulses to the heart, thus causing her symptoms. I then referred her to a fine surgeon who removed the needle.

Her symptoms cleared up completely. Nothing more

was ever done. Needless to say, she was grateful, even though I never adjusted her spine. The interference to the flow of impulses had been cleared when the needle was removed.

Later, while talking about how the needle might have entered her body, she recalled a likely incident. Her mother was a seamstress. It was her mother's habit of sticking the unused needles in a pad near her work rather than in a pincushion. When the young lady was about twelve years of age, she bumped into this pad of needles. One entered her upper arm. It was never found again until I located it during her spinal checkup. Evidently, the needle coasted around her body coming to rest in that dorsal area of her spine. After the needle was removed, allowing the nervous system to function normally, she enjoyed health once more.

May I relate another experience: A young girl was brought into my office. Her condition was diagnosed as epilepsy by medical doctors. Medication prescribed did not help. The convulsions persisted. Could I be of help?

At first thought, one may not associate this type of a health problem with the nervous system and with spinal subluxations.

Spinal analysis located the vertebra which was causing the problem. The vertebra was subluxated and was causing an interference on the nervous system. Spinal adjustments released the interference on the nervous system and allowed a normal impulse energy flow from the brain to the body. In a short time, the convulsions entirely ceased and have never recurred.

Diagnosed medically as having epilepsy, this young lady later married and raised her family. The last time I visited with her parents, they informed me that she was employed at a local bank and enjoying good health.

Though certainly it is not the answer to all epilepsy cases, chiropractic certainly deserves consideration in these cases. Nerve pressure or interference due to subluxated vertebrae may well be a primary cause in some epilepsy cases. Chiropractic is most certainly not a cure-all. Chiropractic adds nothing to the body nor does it take anything away. Chiropractic releases pressures or interferences from the nervous system through spinal adjustments. Health restoration comes from within when the nervous system is free to carry its normal impulse energy supply from brain to body and body back to brain.

One might wonder how nerve interference could cause such a problem and how the release of the nerve interferences could result in a return to health. Chiropractic offers this explanation. A subluxation causes an interference with nerves supplying the kidneys. This causes a malfunction of the kidneys. The kidneys' role in eliminating body waste is not carried on in a normal manner.

When the poisons or toxins in the blood stream have reached a dangerous level, a convulsion takes place. This convulsion is literally to detoxify the toxin or poison being carried by the circulatory system. In the convulsion, violent contraction takes place. The body thus burns up the poisons which have accumulated by the process of the violent muscular action. When the toxins reach a level which is no longer dangerous, the convulsions cease until the arrival of any future accumulation which is dangerous to the body. At that time convulsions recur.

When spinal adjustments release the interference on

the nerves to the kidneys, normal function returns. As normal function returns, the convulsions cease.

Experiences similar to these are recounted daily in the thousands of chiropractic offices that are devoted to the practice of chiropractic confined within its own principles.

People who suffer from headaches may benefit from the following history of this man.

The patient was a man in his fifties. He told me that, chronically, his head ached so much that to gain relief there were times when he literally pounded his head against a wall. Hard to believe, but true!

He described his experience: Some years before, while attending a church outing at the ocean, he was standing on a large log near the surf. He did not see a big breaker wave coming. Before he knew what happened, the log was on top of him and other people were pulling at his legs to get him out from under it. He says his friends almost pulled his head off to get him out from under the log.

In a short while, headaches developed. As time went on, they became more severe. He tried everything and every doctor he heard of who might help him. None did. He was in my office with his problem.

I checked his neck. It was so sore to touch it made him cry out. He had been living with this condition for years.

Analysis of the cervical spine revealed the atlas or first vertebra was severely subluxated. I hesitated to adjust him, but nevertheless I did.

Although he did not recover completely from his pains, he did have a marked lessening of pain, and he enjoyed much better health than before. Evidently, too much damage had been done at the time of his accident for a complete recovery. Accidents such as these are extremely dangerous.

Many people have asked this question many times: How many symptoms can be caused, and how many different organs of the body can be affected by spinal subluxations?

For the answer, I turn to the late H. C. Chance, D.C., PhC, Professor of Neurology from the Palmer School of Chiropractic. He is a leading neurologist in his field. His conclusion was: "Clinically, a pressure in the region of the Atlas and Axis may affect any or all functions.[1]"

Following an accident, it is vitally important for an individual to have the spine checked for the presence of subluxated vertebrae (vertebrae out of normal position causing pressure or interference on the nervous system). The spine is the field of chiropractic.

Many people simply do not understand or appreciate the vital role that the spine plays in health and sickness. But an understanding of this role is necessary to appreciate the science of chiropractic.

Hippocrates, the Father of Healing once wrote:

"It is most necessary to know the nature of the spine, what its natural purposes are, for such knowledge will be a requisite for many diseases.[2]"

Further, Hippocrates said:

"One or more vertebrae of the spine may or may not go out of place very much. They might give way very little, and if they do, they are likely to produce serious complications, and even death, if not properly adjusted.

It appears to me that one ought to know what diseases arise in men, from the powers and what from the structure. By powers I mean intense and strong juices, and by structures, whatever confirmations there are in men. The spinal marrow if it did not break it, and if compressed and strangled, it would induce insensibility of many great and important parts. Many diseases are related to the spine.[3]"

Chiropractic is the philosophy, science and art concerned with the detection, location and adjustment of vertebral subluxations in the spinal column. Included in the practice of chiropractic are the use of the x-ray and other analytical instruments to determine the presence or absence of nerve interference and vertebral subluxations.

The practice of chiropractic demands that very precise scientific methods be used in determining the presence of and the adjusting of subluxated vertebrae. Equally important are exacting methods to determine if the nerve interference or pressures have been released by spinal adjustment.

Chiropractic is not a hit-or-miss practice, nor is it a bone-cracking profession. Neither is it concerned with spinal manipulation or with orthopedic, manipulative therapeutics. Indeed, chiropractic is none of these. Rather, chiropractic is an EXACT, specific practice to adjust vertebrae which are subluxated and causing an interference on the nervous system. EXACT means are also used to determine if the interference on the nervous system has been released.

In June, 1985, **Upper Cervical Monograph** published by the National Upper Cervical Chiropractic Association,

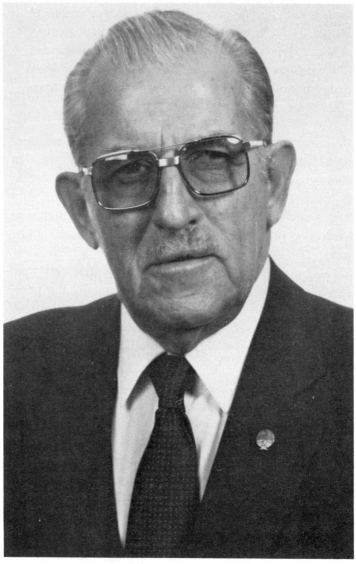

Ralph R. Gregory, D.C.

Inc.,* Ralph R. Gregory, D.C., an ardent researcher in chiropractic, writes:

> "Getting well involves more than getting relief from symptoms. Chiropractially, it involves correction of the bodily distortions and reduction or correction of the misalignment factors of the subluxation. When these two factors are corrected and proven by measurement, the chiropractor should feel confident that he was responsible for helping the patient.
>
> The subluxation stabilizes only when the misalignment factors are sufficiently reduced and the vertebral facets are in proper apposition. If misalignments are increased, greater loss of articulatory alignment occurs and greater loss of vertebral function. How, then, can a patient be benefitted by an increased misalignment? Vertebral misalignment is an abnormal state in the spinal column. Normal vertebral function requires the alignment of the vertebrae to the vertical axis of the body. The organization and form of vertebrae is such that alignment is a pre-requisite to normal vertebral function. Vertebrae are structured to be in a normal position.[4]"

James W. Young, D.C.,** a chiropractic researcher involved in research in spinal adjusting states his opinion:

> "A chiropractic adjustment is a very exacting procedure. The proper adjustment releases the spinal cord, nerve fiber, interference present in the occipito-atlanto-axial (occiput, atlas, axis) region of the spine caused by the vertebral subluxation. A normal impulse flow is restored over the nervous system.[5]"

----

* National Upper Cervical Chiropractic Association, headquarters, Monroe, Michigan. World-wide membership dedicated to research in spinal analysis and adjusting.

** James W. Young, D.C., a pioneer researcher involved in the development and application of instrumentation for specific, scientific, spinal adjusting. Sunnyvale, Calif.

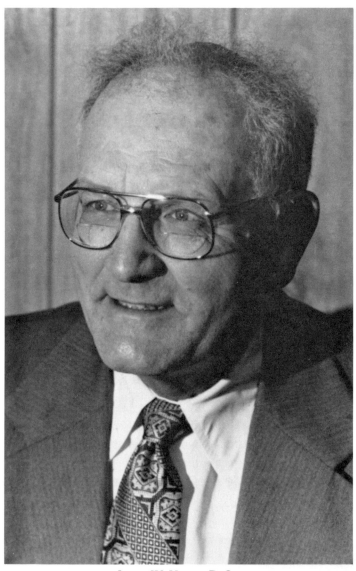

James W. Young, D.C.

But the demands of chiropractic are not limited to knowledge of exacting procedures. Chiropractic also demands thorough understanding of spinal anatomy and of spinal functions. From the book, **Chiropractic Anatomy**, by Mabel Heath Palmer, D.C., PhC., one finds this concise description:

> The spine, improperly called the backbone, is formed of a series of bones called vertebrae (turning bones), a single one being a vertebra. The number in early life is 33, but in adults there are only 26 vertebrae, for the sacrum and coccyx become fused into single pieces. There are 24 permanently movable vertebrae. The total number of 33 segments are grouped as follows: 7 cervical vertebrae (pertaining to cervix, neck), 12 dorsal vertebrae (back), 5 lumbar vertebrae (loin), 5 segments in the sacrum and 4 segments in the coccyx. In the adult, the 5 pieces in the sacrum become fused together and so also do the 4 pieces in the coccyx; they are, therefore, then classified as one sacrum and one coccyx. The 24 vertebrae are called the movable or the true vertebrae; the sacrum and the coccyx are immovable or false vertebrae.
>
> A spinal column is pyramidal in shape, the base downward and the apex formed by the superior portion. It is usually one-third of the height of the individual, being about two feet and two, or three, inches in length. All animals known as vertebrata have a spine like mans': for example, mammals, birds, reptiles and fishes. Those forms of life known as the invertebrata, such as the mollusk, the oyster, and the snail, have no spines, but such structural formation as is adapted to the life of their kind.
>
> The spine has four curves, two primary and two secondary curves. The primary curves are the dorsal and the pelvic. The

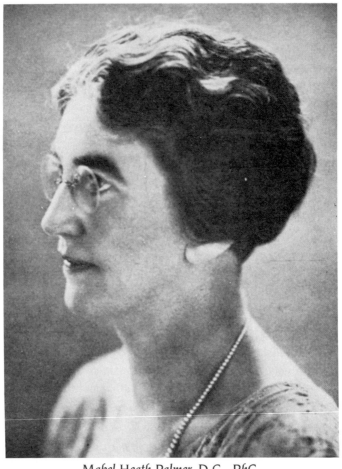

Mabel Heath Palmer, D.C., PhC.

secondary are the cervical and lumbar curves. The dorsal curve extends from the second dorsal vertebra to the twelfth dorsal vertebra, the pelvic curve extends from the sacro-vertebral angle to the coccyx, and both these curves are maintained even in the supine position. The cervical curve extends from the second cervical vertebra to the second dorsal vertebra, the lumbar curve extends from the twelfth dorsal vertebra to the sacro-vertebral angle. These curves are called secondary because they are brought into use immediately when one assumes an upright position. The spinal column forms a single support for the head and trunk, and is a strong-walled canal guarding the spinal cord. It is the central line-shaft of man, it holds the body erect, and is the base from which the trunk muscles act. It permits of all motion such as flexing, extension, rotation and counter extension.[6]

The functions of the spine are many. Mainly, these functions can be found as serving part of the body's framework, serving for attachment of muscles allowing for movement and motion, and surely one of the most important functions is the transmission and protection of the spinal nerves and spinal cord as messages are carried to and from the brain.

Further quoting from **Chiropractic Anatomy** by Mabel Heath Palmer, D.C., PhC.:

''*The brain...is the seat of all intelligence in the body, the habitat of Innate Intelligence, which is the director of all functions in the body, from the time of birth to the dissolution of the physical and mental, which is death. The brain is the place from which the mental currents, which control all functions of the body, emanate and flow to all parts of the body, to each tissue cell, the brain constitutes the beginning and the ending of the one great cycle called life.*[7]"

In his book **Anatomy Of The Human Body**, Henry Gray, F.R.S., explains the relationship between the brain and the spinal column.

"*The brain is usually described as consisting of three main divisions, namely; hind-brain, mid-brain and fore-brain. The hind-brain is usually sub-divided into medulla oblongata, pons and cerebellum. The medulla oblongata extends from the spinal cord to the lower margin of the pons. A plane passing transversly below the pyramidal decussation and above the first pair of cervical nerves corresponds with the upper border of the atlas behind, and the middle of the odontoid process of the axis in front; at this level the medulla oblongata is continuous with the medulla spinalis (spinal cord).*[8]"

Further quoting:

"*The medulla spinalis or spinal cord forms the elongated, nearly cylindrical, part of the central nervous system which occupies the upper two-thirds of the vertebral canal. Its average length in the male is about 45 cm., in the female from 42 to 43 cm., while its weight amounts to about 30 gms. It extends from the levels of the upper border of the atlas to that of the lower border of the first, or upper border of the second, lumbar vertebra. Above, it is continuous with the brain; below, it ends in a conical extremity, the conus medullaris, from the apex of which a delicate filament, the filum terminale descends to the first segment of the coccyx.*[9]"

Certainly, it is becoming apparent that the brain, the spinal column and the spine are extremely complicated. They are also very fragile. They can and often do survive severe blows and strains. But, obviously, there are limits to what they can take. The spinal column has its limits.

If we study the spinal column, we find that the vertebrae or spinal bones below the second cervical or neck vertebrae are very limited in their individual movement or range-of-motion. This range-of-motion is limited by intervertebral discs between each vertebra. These discs hold the vertebrae apart and yet together. Muscles and ligaments also control the range-of-motion as do the superior and inferior articular or bony processes on each vertebra.

With their limited range-of-motion, the spinal bones below the second cervical vertebra are not capable of becoming misaligned far enough to become subluxated. However, these same spinal bones may become misaligned due to abnormal muscle relaxation or contraction.

To appreciate this fact and to understand or visualize what is meant by "limited range-of-motion", consider one of our many inventions patterned after the body structures; the ordinary zipper. Here we find movement by many partially locked pieces of metal, each held together, yet each having a range-of-motion. The whole unit has a range-of-motion controlled by each segmental motion.

Except the two topmost vertebrae, the spine, too, is interlocked by bony processes. These restrict the movement of each individual bone yet allow movement for the structure as a whole. The atlas vertebra is held by muscles and ligaments only. The axis vertebra is held by muscles, ligaments, and inferior articular processes.

The following from **Chiropractic Anatomy** by Mabel Heath Palmer, D.C., should provide a better comprehension of these bones and their articulations:

1. *The Atlanto-axial Articulation (atlas and axis) is a diathrodial joint (a diathrodial joint is a joint with gliding motion and which is freely movable), and is subclassed as an arthrodial and pivot joint (an arthrodial joint is an articulation or joint which allows a gliding motion of the surfaces. Pivot refers to a turning joint).*

2. *The Occipito-Atlanta (occiput-atlas) is a diathrodial joint and also a ginglymoarthrodial and condyloid joint, (ginglymo refers to a hinged joint). (Arthrodial refers to an articulation or joint which allows a gliding motion of the surfaces). Condoloid, refers to resembling eminence at the articular end of a bone). The Occipito-axial Articulation (occiput-axis) is diathrodial.*[10]

If either or both of the upper two vertebrae become locked out of their normal range-of-motion and become subluxated, an interference or pressure is made on the brain stem or the spinal cord at the level of the subluxation.

As the spinal cord exits from the skull, it passes through the spinal canal. At the level of the first and second cervical vertebrae, the spinal cord is composed of trillions of nerve fibers carrying a flowing energy from the brain to the body. This collection of nerve fibers could be compared to the main cable in a wiring system before distribution. The spinal cord at this level is an extension of the brain before any major divisions take place on the nervous system. It is not difficult to understand that pressure on the spinal cord due to a subluxated first or second vertebra could interrupt the energy impulse flow between the brain and body, in turn causing many health problems. This results in abnormal function in the tissues or organs affected by the interrupted or decreased impulse supply.

When there is a subluxation, normal bodily functions cannot be restored until the nerve impulse flow from brain to body is restored. The subluxated vertebra or vertebrae must be adjusted to release the interference or pressure on the spinal cord. When the impulse flow is once more re-established normal function returns to bodily tissues and organs provided that reparation can be accomplished. The body heals itself from within.

This healing is an innate function and activity which in no way or manner can be duplicated from an outside source. Chiropractic recognizes this innate healing quality within each individual.

Usually, a subluxation is the result of an invasionary force, a fall, an accident, (a strain or blow), which overcomes the internal, resistive force of the spine and forces a vertebra to exceed its normal range-of-motion. The vertebra becomes locked out-of-position due to muscle contraction. The antagonistic muscle is unable to exert its normal pull and, thus, balance the vertebra into its normal position or range. A subluxation is present when a vertebra is out-of-juxtaposition with the vertebra above it or the vertebra below it, or both and causing an interference or pressure on nerves.

How are the uppermost two bones in the neck region of the spine different from the rest of the vertebrae? Unlike other vertebrae, no bony or osseous locks are present except the inferior articular processes of axis.

Their range-of-motion is, thus, much greater than the other spinal bones.

The first or topmost vertebra is called the Atlas vertebra. It takes its name from the early Grecian scholars. I have read that the Greeks called it Atlas because it held up the world—the head representing the most important anatomical part. Even today, we see ancient statues of "Atlas" with one hand extended to hold up the world. To the Greeks, the atlas vertebra must have been all-important.

The second vertebra or axis, the pivot upon which the atlas vertebra rotates was named Epistropheus by the Greeks.

Today, these two vertebra are equally as important as they seem to have been in the time of the ancient Greeks. Unfortunately, there are times when this importance is overlooked.

I have reached a conclusion about "why" the first two cervical vertebrae are held only by ligaments and muscles rather than by bony locks to restrict their range-of-motion except the inferior articular processes of axis.

A subluxation can occur when the invasionary, external force overcomes that internal resistance force within our bodies. Just as a bone can be fractured when such force enters the body and there is no "give" in the structure, so can a subluxation occur in the spine when external forces enter the body. The uppermost two vertebrae are literally the safety factors in the spine protecting the spinal cord from damage as it emits from the skull. Their range-of-motion is much greater than the other spinal bones. External forces entering the body are transmitted to the spine. Being segmented, it absorbs these outside forces. Most of the time these external, invasionary forces are dissipated, and no harm is done.

If, however, the forces invading the body are too great, the range of vertebral movement of the two topmost vertebrae may be extended beyond the normal range. Due to muscle contraction they may be locked out of their normal range of motion. Interference is made on the nervous system at the level of the subluxated vertebrae. The subluxation occurs in the upper cervical or neck area. The uppermost two vertebrae, the atlas and axis vertebrae, are the most important in the process of absorbing invasionary forces entering the body.

Picture, if you will, the soft, delicate spinal cord passing from our solid bony skulls into the segmented shaft of 24 spinal bones. Because of their range-of-movement the atlas and axis vertebrae are the safety factor in every spine. With their range-of-movement, these two bones protect the spinal cord from injury. In many instances, they act as a safety valve against forces entering the body. If the uppermost vertebrae were secured by bony locks, ''species vertebrata'' would, in my opinion, have ceased to exist long ago.

Some years ago, the chiropractic profession did a survey to assess the existence of subluxations in different age groups. Surprisingly, the survey revealed that between 80 and 85 percent of spinal subluxations were present in children under the age of twelve years. The next five to eight percent were present in adults up to the age of 25 years. The next five to ten percent were present in individuals over 25 years of age.

This indicated that children as well as adults most certainly do need to have their spines checked for nerve interferences. Children's spines should be adjusted when necessary to release spinal interferences. Some of the reasons for subluxation in children include difficult delivery during birth, twists, falls, and tumbles, before the child's muscle structure has strengthened and attained its full tone.

If the nervous system is kept clear of nerve interference during childhood, the individual is, in my opinion, much more likely to grow up as a healthy individual. If, by the same token, interferences are allowed to remain and be present during childhood, the likelihood of illness or poor health is much more likely.

An example of how chiropractic can aid children is in the condition called scoliosis. Scoliosis can occur when the upper vertebrae slip out of their normal sockets or out of their normal articular process. When this happens, the head actually drops lower on one side. Thus the position of the spine is changed. Rather than being centered, the spine must now go into a sideways curve to hold the head erect. If this condition persists, scoliosis develops, i.e., a crookedness of the spine.

School examinations to detect this condition have discovered many cases. Often the victim's parents never suspect the condition of the child. If not corrected, scoliosis can result in a permanent crooked spine. A chronic condition will also produce corresponding changes in the pelvis. One hip will be higher than the other. Leg measurements will also reflect the difference.

Chiropractic can be of definite help in many of these conditions, providing normal bone structures are present in the spine. A chiropractor can help to correct by adjusting the upper spinal bones to their proper position. The head once more assumes its normal articular position. The weight of the head is again centered on the spine where it should normally rest. In this position, the abnormal curvatures are not necessary to hold the head erect and, no longer exist.

Experiences during my many years of practice clearly proved to me that chiropractic can assist the body's defense and recovery systems and alleviate many health problems. I have always felt that if the actual cause of an illness could be found and corrected, that was certainly in the best interest of the patient. And most certainly, finding the actual cause of an illness made much more sense than covering up symptoms with drugs or sedatives.

A spinal check up to determine the presence or absence of vertebral subluxations should, in my opinion, be as common as a medical or dental checkup.

Everyone should know something about the spine. That knowledge would give all people a much better understanding of one of the marvels of the body. It would enable each individual to reason the "how and why" of ill health. When it is understood that every tissue cell, and every organ of the body is connected to and controlled by the brain through the nervous system, then one can more readily grasp the importance of maintaining a spine free of a vertebral subluxation.

Unfortunately, many of us learn about the spine the hard way. Certainly, each of us has known someone who has suffered a fracture of the neck or back. These tragic circumstances require medical or surgical procedures for correction. However, they do make us aware of the importance of the spine and the nervous system. Certainly if injury to the spine brings death or a lasting paralysis, we become even more aware of the spine's importance.

From a chiropractic standpoint, one of the great tragedies is to see an individual who has accidentally injured the spine but fails to have it checked for possible subluxation and adjusted if necessary. Many times chiropractors encounter individuals who have been involved in accidents but have found no bones fractured and no apparent injury. So they do nothing, even though they are, in fact, injured. Months or even years later, symptoms begin to develop as a result of a subluxation and serious health problems may follow. In many instances, this could have been prevented with proper chiropractic care.

However, with extreme divisions within the chiropractic profession, I am well aware that all that is practiced by chiropractors under the name of chiropractic is not chiropractic. The health consumer should exercise extreme care in finding a chiropractor adequately trained to determine the presence or absence of nerve interference due to the spinal subluxation, and who is qualified in spinal adjusting.

References

1. The Subluxation Specific - The Adjustment Specific, B. J. Palmer, D.C., 1934, pg. 171.

2. The Truth About Chiropractic, Dr. R. W. Grim, Dec. 20, 1934, pg. 111.

3. The Truth About Chiropractic, Dr. R. W. Grim, Dec. 20, 1934, pg. 111.

4. The Upper Cervical Monograph, Vol. 3, No. 10, June, 1985, pg. 8.

5. James W. Young, D. C., Sunnyvale, California, a pioneer in the use of instruments in spinal adjusting.

6. Chiropractic Anatomy, Mabel H. Palmer, D. C. PhC., 1923, Vol. IX, Fifth Edition, pg. 44.

7. Chiropractic Anatomy, Mabel H. Palmer, D. C. PhC., 1923, Vol. IX, pg. 405.

8. Anatomy of the Human Body, Henry Gray, F. R. S., 24th Edition, pg. 774, 775.

9. Anatomy of the Human Body, Henry Gray, F. R. S., 24th Edition, pg. 757.

10. Chiropractic Anatomy, Mabel H. Palmer, D. C. PhC., 1923, pg. 92.

CHAPTER III

A HISTORY OF CHIROPRACTIC

Daniel D. Palmer (1845-1913) is the Founder of chiropractic. It was his late-nineteenth-century research into alternative healing techniques that eventually led to the discovery of the principles of this new school of the healing arts. In his book, **The Science Art and Philosophy of Chiropractic**, Palmer relates the history of his discovery on September 18, 1895, in Davenport, Iowa.

"Harvey Lillard, a janitor in the Ryan Block, where I had my office, had been so deaf for seventeen years that he could not hear the racket of a wagon on the street or the ticking of a watch. I made inquiry as to the cause of his deafness and was informed that when he was exerting himself in a cramped, stooped position, he felt something give away in his back and immediately became deaf. An examination showed a vertebra racked from its normal position. I reasoned that if that vertebra was replaced, the man's hearing should be restored. With this object in view, a half-hour's talk persuaded Mr. Lillard to allow me to replace it. I racked it into position by using the spinous process as a lever and soon the man could hear as before. There was nothing accidental about this as it was accomplished with an object in view, and the result expected was obtained.[1]

On many occasions, medical professionals have questioned the believability of Harvey Lillard's hearing restoration through spinal adjustment. Critics note that the acoustic nerve does not leave the cranial vault and, thus, could not be subject to interference from a vertebral subluxation.

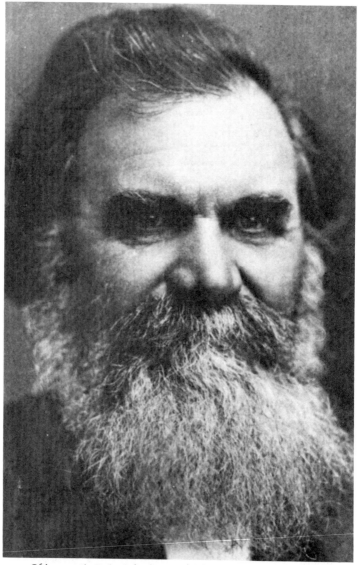

Chiropractic Principle discovered by Daniel David Palmer

The late Dr. Donald O. Pharaoh, Dean of Basic Sciences, Palmer College of Chiropractic, has given this anatomical explanation of how a subluxation affects hearing: "It is anatomically true that the acoustic nerve is located wholly within the cranium. However, there are connections to this nerve from nerves which are situated in areas subject to nerve interference from vertebral subluxations as we know them.[2]" Clinical results since 1895, demonstrate that in many instances the adjustment of subluxations can result in restoration of hearing. (The entire text of Dr. Pharaoh's explanation can be found in the appendices) A.

On many occasions, I had opportunities to dicuss with and listen to Dr. B. J. Palmer tell of the adjustment given to Harvey Lillard by his father, D. D. Palmer. Dr. B. J. Palmer told me that three people were present on that historic occasion: himself, his father, and Harvey Lillard. D. D. Palmer adjusted the axis or second cervical vertebra.

Here is how B. J. Palmer related the details of his father's discovery:

"D. D. Palmer examined Harvey Lillard's spine. He used only his hands, as no instruments were available at that time. In so doing, he discovered an unusually large lump or bump on the back of Lillard's neck. He examined it by pressing with his fingers so he could feel the misalignment better. Harvey told him that the lump had been sore ever since an occasion in which he had popped his neck while in a stooped and cramped position.

D. D. Palmer asked him if he might try to reduce or replace the lump. Harvey Lillard agreed to let him try. Palmer then asked Lillard to lie on the floor face downward. Then

Palmer adjusted the lump in the upper neck area of Harvey Lillard's spine.

Almost instantly, Lillard heard noises of the traffic on the street below and heard D. D. Palmer's voice as he spoke to him. He had been deaf seventeen years."

This was the beginning of the chiropractic profession.

D. D. Palmer discovered that when spinal bones become subluxated or out-of-normal position, the flow of energy or mental impulses over or through the nerves involved is either interrupted or disturbed. Organs or tissues fail to function normally because of the altered impulse flow from the brain to body. Health can be restored from within the body by adjusting the subluxated spinal bones to a normal position, thus releasing the pressure or interference on the nerves which, in turn, re-establishes a normal impulse flow between brain and body, allowing for innate health restoration.

So it was that in 1895 D. D. Palmer discovered that there was an energy or impulse flow over or through the nervous system, and, in fact, it was the vital force within each living body. He also discovered that an interrupted or altered flow of energy from the brain to the body results in an improper function or a lack of function. Palmer called this "dis-ease", i.e., a body not at ease as it is in health.

D. D. Palmer did not have the advantage of using instruments in detecting subluxations. Manual palpation of the spine was the only way to determine if bones were out-of-line. Nevertheless, people soon flocked to Palmer when they heard the miracle he had accomplished for Harvey Lillard.

D. D. Palmer had an inquiring mind about health matters. He had no formal medical education and, for a time, he was a practitioner of magnetic healing. He was always searching for a cause of sickness from within the individual.

Certainly, Palmer was not the first person in history to attempt to adjust the spine. But he is the Founder of Chiropractic. In **The Art Science and Philosophy of Chiropractic**, D D. Palmer wrote:

> *''The basic principle and the principles of chiropractic which have been developed from it, are not new. They are as old as the vertebrata. I have, both in print and by word of mouth, repeatedly stated and now most emphatically repeat the statement, that I am not the first person to replace subluxated vertebra for this art has been practiced for thousands of years. I do claim, however, to be the first to replace displaced vertebrae, by using the spinous and transversed processes as levers wherewith to rack subluxated vertebrae into normal position and from this basic fact, to create a science which is destined to revolutionize the theory and practice of the healing arts.[3]''*

In studying the history and life of D. D. Palmer, one notable feature is the fact that he researched many and any forms of healing prior to his discovery of chiropractic. In his writings, he refers to many individuals and forms of healing that, indeed, looked at the spine whenever they were trying to cure illness.

Palmer frequently refers to others who worked with the spine, but in each instance, he identifies a difference in their procedure as opposed to his. Palmer's precursors manipulated the entire spine. Some cultures used objects to strike the spine, while others walked on the spine in an attempt to regain health. In each instance, these people manipulated the entire spine.

In essence here is how D. D. Palmer described the difference between his discovery and the discoveries of others:

> "*I do not manipulate any portion of the spine. I adjust the subluxated vertebrae by using the spinous and transverse processes as levers. The spinal adjustments I make are direct and specific.*[4]"

It is obvious that it was D. D. Palmer who laid the foundation for the chiropractic profession. His was a totally new idea as to the cause and cure for sickness. This totally new concept was based on the proposition that the cause and cure for sickness was innately within the individual.

It is important to pause and notice here that no medical practice or physical therapy practice is included in D. D. Palmer's concept of chiropractic. D. D. Palmer's concept of chiropractic not only excluded that which is not chiropractic but also included that which is chiropractic. Chiropractic is the adjustment of vertebrae in the spinal column which are out of normal position (subluxated) thus disturbing normal function. He stated, I have created a science of vertebral adjustment.[5]

D. D. Palmer saw the potential of spinal adjusting as so great that '...the science was destined to revolutionize the theory and practice of the healing arts.'

In his book, D. D. Palmer gives this account of how this new science was named:

> "Mrs. Weed, wife of Reverend Samuel Weed of Mon-

mouth, Illinois, and their little daughter took chiropractic adjustments early in 1896, and were much benefitted. Afterwards, Mr. Weed also received adjustments for sciatica. About this time, I asked him to suggest a name in Greek for the science and art which I had created, one which would mean done by hand. Thus originated the word, 'chiropractic'.[6]

The two words which Reverend Samuel Weed put together to make the word chiropractic were: **'Cheir'** *meaning hand and* **'practikos'** *meaning practice.*

At no other time in the history of the healing arts has an idea so sparked people's enthusiasm, imagination, and dedication as did chiropractic. The only desire of these early chiropractic pioneers was a desire to be well and to teach others this new philosophy, science, and art.

As with all great achievements of mankind, each is the product not only of inspiration but also of perspiration. So it was with chiropractic. Actually, D. D. Palmer had studied and researched many forms of healing for about twenty years before his attention finally became focused on vertebral subluxations in the spine. He saw the subluxations as the causative factor of an interruption to the energy flow between the brain and body, thus causing a lack of proper body functions.

Among the various methods he investigated was osteopathy, which was founded in 1874 by A. T. Still. The osteopathic theory held that the cause of disease resulted from an inadequate or improper circulation of blood. This did not answer Palmer's inquisitive mind in its quest for a specific cause of sickness.

He writes:

"In the dim ages of the past when man lived in rude huts

and rocky caves, even up to the present time, he resorted to charms, necromancy and witchcraft for the relief of mental and physical suffering. His whole object was to find an antidote, a specific for each and every ailment which could and would drive out the intruder, as though the disorder was a creature of intelligence. In his desire to free himself from affliction and prolonged existence, he has searched the heavens above, he has gone into the deep blue sea, the bowels of the earth and every portion thereof. He has tried animal and mineral poisons, penetrated the dark forest with superstitious rite and with incantations, has gathered herbs, barks and roots for medicinal use. In his frenzy for relief, trusting that he might find a panacea or at least a specific, he has slaughtered man, beast and bird, making use of their various parts alive and dead. He has made powders, ointments, pills, elixirs, decoctions, tinctures and lotions of all well known vegetables and crawling creatures which could be found, giving therefore his reasons according to his knowledge.[7]*"*

When D. D. Palmer moved to Davenport, Iowa, he was practicing magnetic healing. He continues about his thoughts during this period:

"One question was always uppermost in my mind in the search for the Cause of Disease. I desired to know why one person was ailing and his associate, eating at the same table and working in the same shop at the same bench was not. Why? What difference was there in two persons that caused one to have pneumonia, catarrh, typhoid or rheumatism, while his partner similarly situated, escaped? Why? The question had worried thousands for centuries and was answered in September 1895.[8]*"*

Palmer also recalls other early experiences with spinal adjusting:

> *"Shortly after this relief from deafness (the Harvey Lillard case), I had a case of heart trouble which was not improving. I examined the spine and found a displaced vertebra pressing against the nerves which innervate the heart. I adjusted the vertebra and got immediate relief—nothing accidental or crude about this. Then I began to reason, if two diseases so dissimilar as deafness and heart trouble came from impingement, a pressure on nerves, were not other diseases due to similar cause? Thus the science (knowledge) and art (adjusting) of chiropractic were formed at that time.*
>
> *I founded chiropractic on Osteology, Neurology and Functions—bones, nerves and the manifestations of impulses. I originated the art of adjusting vertebra by using the spinous and transverse process as levers and the knowledge of every principle which is included in the construction of the science of chiropractic.[9]"*

In an attempt to find a cause for sickness, D. D. Palmer had studied for many years. Rather than accepting the theory that sickness was caused by some outside source, he was searching for an internal cause.

Palmer believed that the sole aim of chiropractic is to release any impingements, pressures, or interference on the nervous system caused by subluxated vertebrae. Spinal adjustments allow for a re-establishment of a normal energy impulse flow over or through the nervous system. The innate force within the body heals or restores health from within. The chiropractor neither heals, cures, nor treats. Chiropractic does not fit into the accepted, traditional role of medicine. It is a separate school in the healing arts.

In 1902 D. D. Palmer established a school in Davenport, Iowa to teach the students who came to learn this new work. Most of those who came had benefitted or had their health restored through chiropractic. Between 1909 and 1910, he also started a school in Oregon. Among the first to graduate from the Davenport School was his only son, Bartlett Joshua Palmer, known as B. J. who followed in his father's initiatives and played a major role in the development of the chiropractic profession.

Unfortunately, and quite often in the history of the healing arts, a new idea sparks violent opposition, persecution, and prosecution. This was also true of chiropractic. The early pioneers of chiropractic literally went forth as missionaries. Many were jailed on the charge of practicing medicine without a license. So was D. D. Palmer.

D. D. Palmer and his son B. J. Palmer were arrested in Davenport, Iowa and indicted by a grand jury in 1906, for practicing medicine without a license. D. D. Palmer would not plead guilty to the charge and served time in the Scott County Jail in lieu of paying the fine. Palmer believed that chiropractic was not the practice of medicine. It was a **New and Separate** school in the healing arts. The charge against B. J. Palmer was dismissed. He was neither jailed nor fined. D. D. Palmer wrote:

> "The science of chiropractic has led to the creation of the art of vertebral adjusting. The philosophy of chiropractic (the science and the art) consists of the reasons for the principles which have led up to and the wherefore of vertebral adjusting.
>
> Science refers to that which is to be known; art to that which is to be done; philosophy gives the reasons why of the method and the way in which it is to be performed.

A *science is composed of principles which coincide with mental and physical facts. I have systematized the principles of biology, thereby creating a science. The theory of chiropractic embraces the speculative principles upon which the art of vertebral adjusting is based. The study of chiropractic includes the consideration of the three divisions, viz., the science, art and the philosophy of the two just mentioned.*

Chiropractic to be a science must be specific. In order to be scientific it must contain the knowledge of the principles and facts of biology reduced to an unvarying law and embodied into a system. Where science ends, faith begins. To know the science of chiropractic is to have a knowledge of the principles which compose it. The ability to put that knowledge into practice is chiropractic art.

To know chiropractic as a science, we must become familiar with its principles, we must make it scientific. To know it as an art is to make it specific, make use of the knowledge which composes the science. A chiropractor is one who has a knowledge of the science and art of chiropractic, one who is capable of performing the art of adjusting vertebrae; he should, also, comprehend the philosophy of the science and art, the reasons for so doing.[10]*"*

When D. D. Palmer passed away in 1913, he had given the world the philosophy, science, and art of a new school in the healing arts. His work was also destined to cause the other healing professions to "look within" for the cause of many of the ills of mankind. The unexplored territory of the spine would never be the same. A new era in spinal research was ushered in by that spinal adjustment which restored the hearing of a man who waited in silence for seventeen years.

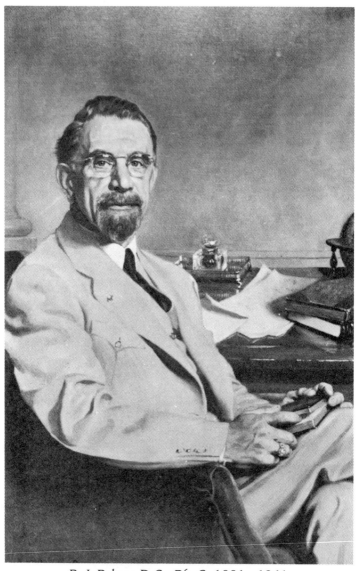

B. J. Palmer, D.C., Ph. C. 1881—1961

It must be recalled that in the beginning, chiropractic was unknown. No knowledge of it existed. There was no profession. No legislation existed granting licensure. No legal decisions upholding chiropractic as a separate school in the healing arts had been made. Chiropractic was a totally new idea in 1895, as it was moved into the mainstream of the healing professions.

   "Science is knowledge reduced to law and embodied in a system. Science teaches us to know and art to do. The philosophy of a science is the understanding of its principles," wrote D. D. Palmer.[11]*"*

Within this framework was the neophyte chiropractic idea.

Bartlett Joshua Palmer, (1881-1961) son of D. D. Palmer, (better known as B. J.) was destined to have a major, unique role in chiropractic history. There is little question but that B. J.'s genius, dedication, and determination helped chiropractic assume its rightful place in the healing arts. Had he not done so, the chiropractic idea and profession undoubtedly would not exist today.

Dr. Mabel Heath Palmer, wife of Dr. B. J. Palmer, was also most instrumental in furthering the profession. She attended Rush Medical College and, upon graduation, taught anatomy at the Palmer School of Chiropractic for many years. Her book, **Chiropractic Anatomy** is still used as a text and reference.

In 1936 I enrolled as a student at the Palmer School of Chiropractic. I was fortunate to have Dr. B. J. Palmer as my instructor in chiropractic philosophy and technique.

Dr. B. J. Palmer was also in charge of the famous B. J. Palmer Chiropractic Research Clinic, which opened in

1935. In his clinic, researchers scientifically established the ability of vertebral adjustments to restore the flow of energy or mental impulse over the nervous system following adjustment. Laboratory tests proved that changes took place in the body following spinal adjusting. The research included use of instruments to analyze spinal temperature differentials, impulse flow over the nervous system, spinal x-rays, and various laboratory tests.

One very important development in the history of chiropractic was the use of the x-ray. The x-ray has played a vital role in chiropractic practice by helping locate spinal subluxations.

The first x-ray picture ever made of a human spinal column was taken by Dr. B. J. Palmer and his associates in 1910. It was not until that year that an x-ray machine was manufactured which had sufficient power to penetrate the spinal column or go through the thickness of the body necessary to make these pictures.

As soon as this machine was created, Dr. B. J. Palmer ordered one and then set up a complete x-ray laboratory at the Palmer School. Research began with advent of the use of the x-ray, which, in Dr. Palmer's words, "was destined to revolutionize the practice of chiropractic from a hit-and-miss method to one of exactitude and scientific precision."

In 1925, Dossa Evins, an electrical engineer and later a student at the Palmer School conceived the idea of an instrument to locate the vertebral subluxations of the spine by measuring the heat differentials caused by interferences to the impulse or energy flow over or through the nervous system. The instrument he invented was named the neurocalometer.

The neurocalograph is yet another chiropractic instrument. It records and graphs heat differentials on the sides of the spine. It does this by using Dossa Evins' method of determining the heat differentials. Otto Schiernbeck, an electrical engineer, invented the neurocalograph with the help and advice of Dr. B. J. Palmer. The neurocalograph records the temperature differential, helping to determine the presence or absence of a subluxation in the spine.

The electroencephaloneuromentimpograph* was a research instrument used to determine and record nerve force flow before and after spinal adjustments. Each patient in the B. J. Palmer Chiropractic Research Clinic was checked bi-weekly to record the energy flow over the nervous system following spinal adjustment. This bi-weekly checkup validated the theory put forth by D. D. Palmer that a subluxated vertebra interrupted the energy flow over the nervous system and that a normal flow of energy was restored following spinal adjustment.

Precision spinal x-rays also showed that the vertebra assumed a normal re-alignment following proper spinal adjustment.

The B. J. Palmer Chiropractic Research Clinic used these instruments and, validated the discovery of D. D. Palmer that energy flows efferently (outward nerve impulses flowing from the brain to body) over the nervous system and afferently (inward nerve impulses flowing from the body to the brain). Subluxated vertebrae

------

* This instrument, the electroencephaloneuromentimpograph, measures, evaluates and calibrates the quantity flow of mental impulse flow from brain to body, both before and after spinal adjustment.

can interfere with this energy flow. Spinal adjustments correct the vertebral subluxation. This allows for an increased or a normal energy flow over the nervous system.

The B. J. Palmer Chiropractic Research Clinic was the first and finest research institution in the history of chiropractic. I was privileged to intern in this clinic. Most unfortunately, it was disbanded following the death of Dr. B. J. Palmer in 1961. His research did much to demonstrate the authenticity of chiropractic.

I first met Dr. B. J. Palmer in 1936. I worked with him in many capacities in the International Chiropractors Association, serving as a member of the Board of Control from 1951 until his passing in 1961. During these years, he was the President of the organization. Later, when I served as President of the International Chiropractors Association, my experiences with B. J. proved invaluable to me. I was able to direct programs for chiropractic acceptance in many areas such as insurance, Union Health and Welfare contracts, Federal Employees Health Benefit Plans, and Medicare.

Dr. B. J. Palmer led the effort necessary to establish chiropractic legally as a separate school in the healing arts. Over the years, many legal battles ensued, wherein chiropractors were charged with practicing medicine without a license. These challenges were the occasions for chiropractors to prove in court that chiropractic has its own philosophy, science, and art, in turn, meeting the requirements essential for a separate school.

One cannot fully comprehend the full importance of chiropractic being a separate school in the healing arts unless one is familiar with the landmark legal decision which established the legal guidelines necessary for a separate school. The legal decision that designated the meaning of "separate school" happened in 1888, with **Nelson vs Harrington, 72, Wisconsin 591, 40 N.W. 228 (1888)**, I feel an understanding of this landmark case is so germane to the issue of a separate school that I have reproduced the entire text of the ruling in the appendix, (see Appendix). However, the pertinent portions follow below. A 1

To better understand the importance of Nelson vs Harrington, it is important to know that this was the first case in U.S. legal history which decided what had to be proven to constitute a school of medicine. The decision in Nelson vs Harrington is the basis of all law on the subject of different schools of medicine and is quoted and followed everywhere.

To have a separate school in the healing arts, the courts have stated that the school must have rules and principles of practice which all of its members profess to follow. Chiropractic fits this definition. Chiropractic is a recognized school of healing with its own art, science, and philosophy of disease. Chiropractic is a theory separate and distinct and capable of being identified and bounded within its own principles and practice.

In the case of Nelson vs Harrington, Thomas Nelson (then about 15 years of age) was afflicted with a disease of his right hip jont. Harrington was a physician, practicing in Madison, Wisconsin. Rather than treating the patient as a physician and using the ordinary skill and care as is ordinarily exercised by physicians, Harrington treated the boy in a manner of a clairvoyant physician.

Thus the case of Nelson vs Harrington was an action brought to recover damages of the alleged malpractice of the defendant (Harrington) as a physician.

The following are pertinent quotes from the legal decision in **Nelson vs Harrington 72 Wisconsin 591, 40 N.W. 228 (1888):**

> ''*The defendant is what is known as a clairvoyant physician, and held himself out, as other physicians do, as competent to treat diseases of the human system. He did not belong to, or practice in accordance with the rules of, any existing school of physicians governed by formulated rules for treating diseases and injuries, to which rules all practitioners of that school are supposed to adhere. The testimony shows that his mode of diagnosis and treatment consisted in voluntarily going into a sort of trance condition, and while in such condition to give a diagnosis of the case and prescribe for the ailment of the patient thus disclosed. He made no personal examination, applied no tests to discover the malady, and resorted to no other source of information as to the past or present condition of the plaintiff. Indeed, he did not profess to have been educated in the science of medicine. He trusted implicitly to the accuracy of his diagnosis thus made and of his prescriptions thus given.*
>
> *The general rule above stated requires of one holding himself of as a physician* **the exercise of the same skill and care as is ordinarily exercised by physicians in good standing who belong to the same school of medicine and practice under the same rule. To constitute a school of medicine under this rule, it must have rules and principles of practice for the guidance of all its members, as respects principles, diagnosis, and remedies, which each member is supposed to observe in any given case.** (Bold

italics, mine). Thus, any competent practitioner of any given school would treat a given case substantially the same as any other competent of the same school would treat it. One school may believe in the potency of drugs and blood-letting, and another may believe in the principle **similia similibus curantur;** *still others may believe in the potency of water, or of roots and herbs; yet each school has its own peculiar principles and rules for the government of its practitioners in the treatment of diseases.*[12]''

The decision of Nelson vs Harrington drew the lines around each profession which purports to be a separate school in the healing arts.

Here is how the decision relates directly to chiropractic: To be a separate school in the healing arts, chiropractic would need its own, unique principles and practice. Clearly, that is what D. D. Palmer gave chiropractic. The principles involved in spinal adjusting clearly constitute a separate school of medicine.

But here is a vital point, **Vis a Vis,** the current 'mixer' philosophy of chiropractic:

To add other practices to chiropractic such as medical or physical therapy practices, violates the principles which separate chiropractic from other schools in the healing arts. To invade other professional practices under the guise of chiropractic is to abandon the right to be judged by one's peers and by one's patients in cases of malpractice.

When the right and the duty to be judged by one's peers is lost, it is difficult to maintain a separate profession in the healing arts. Further, intrusion into other professional practices without proper training poses a very real danger to the public. It is through behavior such as this, that quackery flourishes.

Another important figure in the history of chiropractic is Mr. Arthur T. Holmes, an attorney in the firm of Morris, Winter, Esch and Holmes. In 1924, Holmes wrote a book entitled **Malpractice As Applied To Chiropractors.** Mr. Holmes' book did much to establish and to advance chiropractic as a separate, distinct school. Holmes served as the national counsel for the Universal Chiropractors Association in close association with Dr. B. J. Palmer. In his book, Holmes had this to say about Nelson vs Harrington:

> *"...from the malpractice viewpoint there are the following schools of medicine:*

> 1. *Allopath*
>
> 2. *Homeopath*
>
> 3. *Christian Science*
>
> 4. *Eclectic*
>
> 5. *Thompsonian*
>
> 6. *Osteopathic*
>
> 7. *Chiropractic (which for the purposes of malpractice is classed as a school of medicine)*

> *Now bear in mind that all of these systems are separate and distinct and the reader immediately asks: "How are they separate and how does the court determine what is a school?"*

The issues that determine the guidelines for a separate and distinct school were determined by Nelson vs Harrington. But Holmes' explanation of what constitutes a separate school is direct and to the point.

"This (the issue of a separate school) was decided in a basic case which is reproduced in whole in this book—**Nelson vs Harrington, 72 Wisconsin, 591 40 N.W. 228 (1888).** This was a case of a clairvoyant physician. The rule laid down in that case is that to constitute a recognized school of medicine there must be a theory of principles and practices concerning disease, the diagnosis, and remedy, which all the members of the school profess and are required to follow. This means that there must be some theory concerning disease or the cause thereof.

Now what does 'diagnosis' mean from the angle of the court in determining whether there is a separate school or not? 'Diagnosis' means finding out what is wrong with the patient or "what is causing the disease according to the above theory of disease."

In the chiropractic theory this would be by palpation, x-ray, nerve tracing, etc. In the Allopathic school, it would be to give a medical name to a group of symptoms or a condition.

Now, although spinal analysis is different from medical diagnosis, the courts have held it really means finding what is wrong with the patient according to the school or theory of disease.

These further quotes from Attorney Holmes help clarify:

In determining whether there is a separate school, what does the court mean when it speaks of the remedy? It does not necessarily mean medicine but it means whatever that school uses or does to restore the patient to health or eliminate the cause of disease.

With the allopath physician it would be whatever medicine was prescribed or surgical operation performed and with the Christian Scientists whatever was done to correct the spiritual error. In chiropractic it would be the adjustment of the articulations of the spine.

These principles above enumerated must be professed and followed by the members of that school."

To quote Holmes further:

"Chiropractic is now a science unto itself. It is separate and distinct from allopathic medicine and from osteopathy, or any form or system of healing. It has its own particular methods of ascertaining the cause of disease, and its own particular means of eliminating the cause and allowing innate to restore the patient to health.[13]"

Attorney Holmes accomplished a great deal in the legal field which aided the establishment of chiropractic as a separate school in the healing arts.

In the chapter **Chiropractic and the Law**, I have included other legal decisions for further clarification and have included substantiation that chiropractic is a separate practice.

Chiropractic was challenged in state after state and always the charge was practicing medicine without a license: But under the strong uncompromising leadership of Dr. B. J. Palmer, chiropractic proved itself to be a separate, distinct practice in the healing profession. Dr. B. J. Palmer's leadership helped validate the theory of chiropractic as defined by D. D. Palmer.

An interesting book on the history of chiropractic is **The Evolution of Chiropractic**, by A. August Dye, D. C. This book records the many challenges to chiropractors in which they were accused of practicing medicine without a license.

"...1911-1914, we find the medical associations and the prosecuting agents very active, and, as well, quite successful in securing convictions. The campaign against chiropractic was most active in Montana, Wyoming and California. It was also hot and heavy in Ohio, Indiana and Kansas. Where the defining clause of the practice act was most stringent, or the criminal code prevented jury trials, leaving the trial judge in control, himself usually with the 'educated' medical persecution and against the 'ignorant, untutored' chiropractor, we find frequent convictions, with the 'convict' sentenced to a term in jail, in some cases as long as six months, accompanied by a threat from the bench if they practiced again on release and brought before it, the next term in durance vile (imprisonment) would be the limit.[14]"

Readily, we can see that if chiropractic had not attained the status as separate in the school of healing arts, chiropractic would have been forced either to gain a medical license or cease and desist from the practice entirely. Obviously, the profession would have been short lived.

To their credit, chiropractors would not plead guilty to practicing medicine without a license. They saw chiropractic as a separate, distinct profession with its own philosophy, science, and art. The decisions gained in these prosecutions led the way for licensing by the separate states, recognition as a separate profession, and the right to be judged by our own peers in case of malpractice.

It is important to note that almost every original state license that was granted for chiropractic was on the basis that chiropractic was a separate, distinct practice, apart from any other profession.

As an example, the Chiropractic Legislative Act of the State of North Carolina defines chiropractic in 90-143 Article as follows:

> "*Definition of Chiropractic: Chiropractic is herein defined to be the science of adjusting the cause of disease by realigning the spine, releasing pressure on nerves radiating from the spine to all parts of the body, and allowing the nerves to carry their full quota of health current (nerve energy) from the brain to all parts of the body.*"

Today, many state legislative bodies are under pressure from those who would enter the back door of medical and physical therapy practices under the guise of chiropractic. So it is that, regretfully, many legislatures have substantially enlarged the scope of practice allowed to the chiropractic profession.

An example of this type of liberal state statute is that found in the Chiropractic Legislative Act in Oregon in 1986, Chapter 684.010, which reads as follows:

> "'*Chiropractic' is defined as that system of adjusting with the hands the articulations of the bony framework of the human body, and the employment and practice of physiotherapy, electrotherapy, hydrotherapy and minor surgery.*"
>
> "*Minor surgery means the use of electrical or other methods for surgical repair and care incident thereto of superficial lacerations and abrasions, benign superficial lesions, and the removal of foreign bodies located in the superficial structures; and the use of antiseptics and local anesthetics, in connection therewith.*"

As one reads the definitions of chiropractic in states like the State of Oregon, it is important to keep in mind that many chiropractic colleges teach many medical and physical therapy practices that have nothing inherent to do with chiropractic. Yet not one of these chiropractic colleges meets the American Medical Association accreditation standards for any of the medical or surgical practices taught. Not one chiropractic college meets the accreditation standards for the practice of physical therapy as adopted by the American Physical Therapy Association.

For example, the 1982 and 1983 Biennial Report of Western States Chiropractic College announced:

> "WSCC *received a federal grant the first ever awarded to a chiropractic college to recruit* Native Americans *into chiropractic. The grant which is distributed through the Federal Health Career Opportunity Program, provides funding for recruitment, financial aid, counseling and study habit assistance.*
>
> *College representatives have been 'on the road' to reach Indian students at reservations, high schools and community colleges in the Northwest. The three year grant totals nearly $225,000 and hopes to recruit 10 to 12 Indian students each year."*

Under the heading "Clinic" in the same publication:

> "*Lab services, phlebotomy,* EKG, *six-hour glucose tolerance test, general chemistries and hematology."*

Further quoting from the publication:

> "*In addition to specialized services in X-ray and Laboratory, the* WSCC *also accepts referrals for consultation, examination, and treatment in the following areas: Routine care, minor surgery, gynecology, physiotherapy, proctol-*

ogy, colonic irrigation, nutrition, counseling, orthotics, (foot levelers), casting.[15]*"

An interesting look back into an intra-professional action that took place in 1965 is most revealing. As President of the International Chiropractors Association, I appointed a committee of three members of my board for a purpose which I felt was most important. They were to meet with a like committee from the other major Chiropractic Association to discuss and, hopefully, arrive at a legally sound and defensible definition and scope of practice for chiropractic so that the profession could ultimately be unified on a separate and distinct definition and scope of practice.

The other Association agreed to my suggestion. They too, appointed a committee of three to meet with ours for the stated purpose. The joint meeting was held in Chicago, Illinois on November 13-14, 1965.

This meeting had the potential of dramatically changing the course of chiropractic for the better. Unfortunately, that was not to be.

After a real, in-depth study of the entire situation, the committee of six agreed to a mutually acceptable definition and scope of practice for the profession. The proposed language excluded methods or practices which were deemed legally to be the practices of other professions.

In a joint statement, both committees from the respective groups reported that they pursued the matter of a legally sound definition, scope of practice, and guidelines for the chiropractic profession. The agreed upon definition and scope of practice by the joint committee is as follows:

"Chiropractic is that Science and Art which utilizes the inherent recuperative powers of the body and deals with the relationship between the nervous system and the spinal column, including its immediate articulations, and the role of this relationship in the restoration and maintenance of health.

The practice of Chiropractic deals with the analysis of any interference with normal nerve transmission and expression, the procedure preparatory to, and complimentary to the correction thereof, by an adjustment of the articulations of the vertebral column and its immediate articulations for the restoration and maintenance of health; it includes the normal regimen and rehabilitation of the patient without the use of drugs or surgery.

The term analysis is construed to include physical examination, the use of x-ray and other analytical instruments generally used in the practice of chiropractic."

Meeting in Hollywood, California on February 21, 1966, the International Chiropractors Association unanimously adopted the definition and scope of practice approved by the joint committee representing the two organizations that had met in Chicago. Ours was the only association to adopt the joint committee recommendations.

Little wonder that a confused public remains in doubt as to the real role of chiropractic. No wonder too, that there is a continued disrespect for the chiropractic profession and a continued, widespread perception of negativism relative to chiropractic. If chiropractic does not have a universally accepted definition and scope of practice and universally accepted standards, chiropractic will not aspire to the public respect that it needs and deserves.

To eliminate the confusion within the profession as to the scope of practice, **A Common, Legally Sound Definition And Scope of Practice Should Be Adopted In All Legislative Jurisdictions, And By The Profession, Making For A Uniform Practice.** Surely those who seek chiropractic care deserve protection from the unqualified practitioners. Those of us who hold chiropractic as a separate philosophy, science and art certainly have no quarrel with state statutes governing chiropractic practice. However, we disagree vigorously with state statute language, which includes medical practices and physical therapy practices as a part of chiropractic. A chiropractor or chiropractic physician who desires to practice medical or physical therapy practices should meet the separate licensing and accreditation standards for these professions. Statute language controlling or defining chiropractic should reflect this requirement.

But, statute language defining chiropractic should not open the back door for unqualified chiropractors to enter the practices of physical therapy and medical practices. In many instances this situation exists at the present time.

The image of chiropractic as a profession has been severely tarnished by this attempt to mix chiropractic with medical or physical therapy practices or with other non-chiropractic, professional practices. What a far cry from the dream and vision of D. D. Palmer when he wrote,

"*No thank you, I do not mix, I give chiropractic straight. If it were mixed with all the methods offered, it would soon lose its identity.*"

''A *chiropractor who comprehends the principles of this science will have no use for adjuncts. Just in proportion as he lacks knowledge and confidence (the two go together) he will use remedies, become a mixer. The more he mixes the less use he has for chiropractic.*[16]''

The early chiropractic pioneers were willing to go to jail for the right to be chiropractors. They wanted to achieve the respect they deserved. Today, their efforts are betrayed by those who mix the art of chiropractic with numerous medical and physical therapy practices.

Dr. B. J. Palmer was the leader of chiropractic through turbulent years of its history. He served as the President of the Chiropractic Health Bureau, which was the forerunner of the International Chiropractors Association. He led the profession in chiropractic legislation, legal matters and other important areas to chiropractic. His writings were voluminous, consisting among other writings, 38 books on chiropractic. He always kept chiropractic confined within its own principles and practices.

In his last published book, **The Great Divide**, Dr. B. J. Palmer writes:

Chiropractic possesses three great, simple fundamentals:

1. *An age-old, yet modern, new principle and practice attaining a new result. An acknowledgement, understanding of, and knowledge of an Internal Innate Intelligence.*

2. *An acknowledgement, understanding of, and knowledge of Interference between Innate and function, between brain and body, creating dis-ease between them.*

3. *An acknowledgement, understanding of, and know-*
   ing how, what, and where and when and why of
   correcting that interference; and permitting a resto-
   ration of flow that balances all normal routines
   between Innate and function, between brain and
   body.[17]

Through the dedicated, determined efforts of Dr. B. J. Palmer, the roots of chiropractic were deepened. The fundamentals of Chiropractic stood the test. The profession grew. In one direction a strong segment of the profession held to the fundamentals propounded by the Palmers. However, in the opposite direction, those of the mixer philosophy pushed forward to usurp practices which were not rightly theirs. Though they failed to meet accreditation standards for practices foreign to chiropractic, the mixer element pushed forward hoping for public acceptance. Chiropractic confined within its own principles was earning a good public reputation. The mixer hid behind that reputation.

Through all of this, the principle and practices of chiropractic remained legally separate and distinct from other professions.

A recent court decision: State of Michigan, Court of Appeals, March 21, 1983, People of the State of Michigan, Plaintiff v James J. Beno, D.C. Defendant, Docket 61368 establishes once again that the scope of chiropractic be kept within the confines of the principles laid down by D. D. Palmer. The pertinent passage of the decision follows:

"*Chiropractors must confine their practice to the location*
and adjustment of vertebral subluxations. Spinal x-rays are

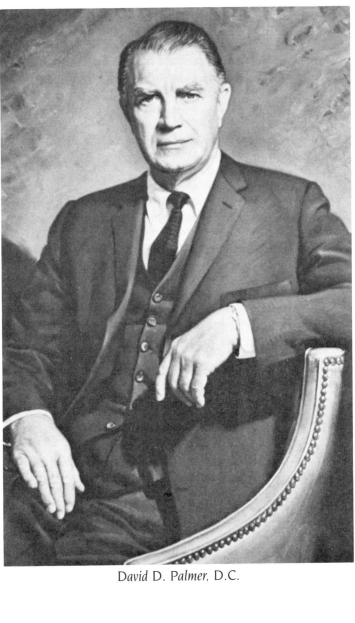

David D. Palmer, D.C.

included. Chiropractors may not render general health or neu-
rological examinations or evaluations, prescribe or dispense
food supplements or vitamins, take x-rays of bodily parts other
than the spinal column, use galvanic current, diathermy, ultra-
sound or other practices included in the practice of physical
therapy.

Neither can a chiropractor in Michigan collect urine speci-
mens, hair specimens or analysis and may not diagnose other
than spinal subluxations or misalignments of the spine.[18]′′

Following an appeal, the Michigan Supreme Court
upheld this decision August, 1985.

David D. Palmer, 1906-1978, was the third generation
of Palmers to lead the profession. He was the grandson
of D. D. Palmer. He came to be known as the Chiropractic
Educator. He carried on the Palmer tradition of upholding chiropractic as a separate philosophy, science, and
art.

Dr. David Palmer ascended to the Presidency of
Palmer College of Chiropractic following the 1961 death
of his father, Dr. B. J. Palmer. Dr. David Palmer and his
wife, Dr. Agnes Palmer were to write further chiropractic
history.

As President of Palmer College of Chiropractic, Dr.
David D. Palmer immediately made changes in the educational areas. He aimed for further acceptance of chiropractic in the educational community and in the
mainstream of the healing arts. He, too, insisted that chiropractic be confined to its own principles and practices
as established by his grandfather and developed by his
father.

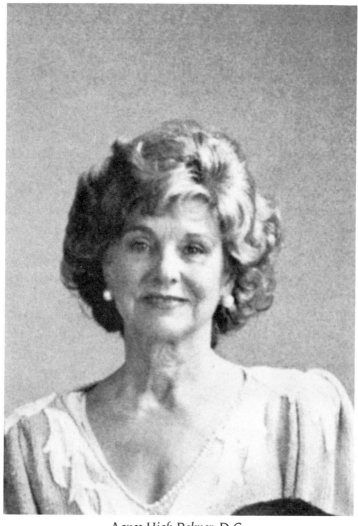

Agnes High Palmer, D.C.

Writing in the preface of his grandfather's book (reprinted from a 1910 edition), Dr. David Palmer clearly states his feelings:

> "My grandfather's work ranks as a most unique and important contribution to the many volumes of literature concerned with the health of humanity. It reveals quite clearly the source and strength of our great profession and in strong tones it says that this incomparable science must never be dissipated, neglected or lost:
>
> No man could have left a finer legacy or a greater challenge to the college he founded and the Palmer College of Chiropractic takes pride in remaining faithful to his inspired principles of Philosophy, Science, and Art. We urge and inspire each and every student to emulate his life's work.[19]"

During his tenure as President of the Palmer College of Chiropractic from 1961 until his death in 1978, Dr. David D. Palmer made many changes on the campus of Palmer College. Among these changes were new buildings and a new auditorium. His aim was "educational excellence" in chiropractic.

It was my pleasure to work closely with Dr. David D. Palmer in the strengthening of the reputation of chiropractic in legislative, legal, and educational arenas. When the Palmer College of Chiropractic gained a non-profit status, I also served on the Board of Trustees until my resignation. Dr. David Palmer added much impetus to further chiropractic as a profession. He passed away in 1978.

The Palmers are the roots of chiropractic. Every chiropractic college and every chiropractor originates from the recognition of the principles of chiropractic as discovered and defined by D. D. Palmer.

Today, chiropractic is known and practiced worldwide. Palmer College of Chiropractic stood as the fountainhead of chiropractic during the years of the Palmers.

And although accreditation may rightly belong in a chapter on education, the impact of accreditation covers a vital era in chiropractic history. Most of the significant history of chiropractic in the recent years, involves and revolves around the accreditation question.

In an address delivered at the Homecoming at Palmer College of Chiropractic in 1969, Dr. David D. Palmer gave this report on progress of accreditation:

"*Now a few words on the matter of securing accreditation for our chiropractic colleges*:

A *number of meetings have been held this past year by several college presidents to develop criteria acceptable to the* U.S. *Office of Education.*

We *have learned that an accrediting agency of our own schools must be free of political association control—completely free. This is the principal reason for the* ACA's *failure to secure acceptance of their accrediting committee. Through no fault of theirs, they represent only a part of the chiropractic educational system and, of course, this same situation prevails with the* ICA. *Washington has continually advised that unilateral efforts are not acceptable. Each separate effort has succeeded only in neutralizing the effectiveness of each other.*

I *believe the proper function of an accrediting agency is to evaluate all schools and not be guilty of trying to gain a political advantage by promoting only a section of our educational system.*

Politics has a legitimate place in our profession—but when it goes so far as to capriciously retard our educational and professional efforts, it should be directed to more profitable ends. Federal accreditation must be left to the school men who know best the college problems. To his everlasting credit, Dr. Leonard Rutherford sees this and has willingly and publicly given the ICA schools his blessings, and without reservation, has encouraged us in our efforts in every possible way. I urge the officials of the ACA to do likewise and, thus, make, as soon as possible, the reality of our own accrediting agency.[20]"

The "number of meetings" referred to in Dr. David D. Palmer's address produced the formation of a new association of colleges known as the Association of Chiropractic Colleges in 1970-71*. This organization of colleges had a prime objective: The formation of a single accrediting agency for recognition by the (U.S.O.E.) United States Office of Education as the accrediting body for the chiropractic profession. For the first time, the majority of chiropractic colleges joined hands in an effort to present a united front in chiropractic education to the United States Office of Education. This effort was spearheaded by Dr. Davd D. Palmer.

Initially, prospects appeared very positive. Progress was made which could produce educational recognition for chiropractic. As Dr. David D. Palmer reported, my action as President of the International Chiropractors

---

* Dr. Ted McCarrel, co-founder of the American College Testing Program (ACT) served as advisor and consultant.

Association had freed the new association of colleges from any political control by the International Chiropractors Association.

However, a similar action did not take place with the other association as Dr. David D. Palmer had urged and hoped for.

In 1971, the (CCE) Council on Chiropractic Education was incorporated. It was now an independent, self-governing organization.

The Superior Court of New Jersey, Appellate Division. A-1121-71: In the matter of the application for approval by Sherman College of Straight Chiropractic, argued November 13, 1978, decided January 5, 1979, wrote this statement in the decision:

> "Again the reason behind the college's lack of accreditation in several other states is its strict adherence to the tenets of the 'straight' school since many of those states require, as a condition to approval, accreditation by **CCE** *which is 'mixing oriented'.*[21]" (Bold italic, mine).

As reported in the **Daily Washington Law Reporter,** January 12, 1981:

> "Sherman College of Straight Chiropractic, et al., vs U.S. Commissioner of Education, et al., Dist Ct., D.C. Civil No 79-2224, July 15, 1980. CCE first applied to the Commissioner for recognition as a reliable authority as to the quality of training offered by chiropractic educational institutions in 1973. An organization called the Association of Chiropractic Colleges (hereinater "ACC") also applied for recognition. ACC was an association representative of several institutions adhering to the 'straight' doctrine. Both applications were denied by the commission."

In 1973, both the (CCE) Council on Chiropractic Education and the (ACC) Association of Chiropractic Colleges failed to gain unilateral accreditation approval by the (U.S.O.E.) United States Office of Education. Following this failure, the colleges entered into a binding arbitration agreement. The agreement was to form one single educational accrediting agency for the purpose of presenting one educational program to the (U.S.O.E) United States Offices of Education. This program was to gain recognition as the accrediting agency for the profession.

> *"The Committee for binding arbitration of the ACC and the CCE met at the Sheraton O'Hare, Rosemont, Illinois, on November 10-11, 1973. The purpose of this meeting was to establish a single accrediting agency for chiropractic education acceptable to the United States Commissioner of Education of the U.S. Office of Education, a division of H.E.W. The following have affixed their signatures only as it relates to their approval of the wording and intent of the binding arbitration contract. The legal acceptance of this contract can only result following acceptance by their respective boards. This document was signed on November 11, 1973, by the Presidents of the ACC, CCE and the college presidents representing the two organizations, as well as other college representatives.[22]"*

In many conferences with officials of the U.S. Office of Education the government officials made it very clear that the U.S. Office of Education was not going to be an arbitrator in a dispute between chiropractic factions. Unless and until the profession could come together in a united educational effort, accreditation would not be realized.

Many conferences with officials of the U.S. Office of

Education confirmed that chiropractic would only be accredited when teaching was confined to the chiropractic principles and practices. As before stated the American Medical Association had accredited all medical practices. The American Physical Therapy Association had already accredited physical therapy. The officials felt that chiropractic should be accredited only if it had a program and teaching leading to the degree of Doctor of Chiropractic (D.C.).

Chiropractors were advised in meetings with educational officials that other allied or "adjunct" programs such as physiotherapy and medical practices should not be included in a chiropractic education and neither should those practices be accredited under a chiropractic accreditation program. Further, the officials gave advice that a chiropractic accrediting agency should confine itself to its own field of training and practice, thus doing the public a service by preparing first-rate chiropractors.

During the period of the binding arbitration between the Association of Chiropractic Colleges, and the Council on Chiropractic Education, the United States Office of Education told the two organizations to get together as one educational effort representing chiropractic education. During this same period, the Council on Chiropractic Education in an unannounced action, submitted its separate standards to the U.S. Office of Education.

Again, I quote from the January 12, 1981, **Daily Washington Reporter:**

"In 1974, CCE *reapplied for recognition and after review of its application, it was recognized.* ACC *however, never reapplied for recognition."*

The intent of the "standards" actually submitted by the Commission on Chiropractic Education is clearly defined.

I quote a paragraph from the Council on Chiropractic Education in the Forward of the Educational Standards:

> " A *Doctor of Chiropractic is a physician concerned with the health needs of the publc as a member of the healing arts. He gives particular attention to the relationship of the structural and neurological aspects of the body in health and disease. He is educated in basic and clinical sciences as well as related health subjects. The purpose of his professional education is to prepare the doctor of chiropractic as a primary health care provider. As a portal of entry to the health delivery system the chiropractic physician must be well-educated to diagnose, including, but not limited to, spinal analysis, to care for the human body in health and disease and to consult with, or refer to, other health care providers. It is this concept of the chiropractic physician which serves as the basis for interpretation of the Educational Standards for Chiropractic colleges.*[23]"

Historically, for many in the chiropractic profession it was then, and still is, most difficult to understand how the same application by the Council on Chiropractic Education denied in 1973, could be approved in 1974.

Lured by educational recognition and by federal funding, many colleges bolted the Association of Chiropractic Colleges, veered sharply toward mixer philosophy, and abdicated their stand to preserve chiropractic within its true concepts as discovered and developed by the Palmers. Selling one's birthright for a "mess of pottage" was, in my opinion, never so real.

The colleges were told by the (CCE) Council on Chiropractic Education that each could maintain its own philosophy of training and teaching but this, too, was a shortlived promise.

It should be clearly understood that the action taken by the U.S. Office of Education in recognizing the Council on Chiropractic Education as an accrediting agency was in no way sponsored by a large segment of the profession. The question still remains, why were the standards in education submitted by the (CCE) Council on Chiropractic Education rejected in 1973, and then accepted in 1974? Particularly is this so when the (CCE) Council on Chiropractic Education was a participant in binding arbitration with the (ACC) Association of Chiropractic Colleges. This arbitration was supposed to arrive at an educational program acceptable to **all** of the educational institutions within the profession. The accreditation issue fostered deeper divisions within the profession.

I believe that it is a gross misuse of the taxpayer's money to educate a chiropractor to practice medical and physical therapy techniques. However, after 1974, the lure of federal dollars outweighed many chiropractic college's commitment to the maintenance of chiropractic as a separate philosophy, science and art. The price many paid was a compromise of their principles. As an example, in an attempt to gain accreditation under the (CCE) Council on Chiropractic Education as well as to qualify some graduates in states requiring or allowing medical or physical therapy practices, the following occurred:

An October, 1977, News Release from the Logan College of Chiropractic (St. Louis, Missouri) reported the following in **World Wide Report**, (a chiropractic magazine):

"*Logan College, anticipating the need for the inclusion of physiotherapy in the Chiropractic curriculum, initiated an elective course in physiotherapy approximately two years ago, in order to meet the criteria of the Council on Chiropractic Education (CCE).*

When the Council on Chiropractic Education met recently in Albuquerque, an amendment to the educational criteria was adopted. This amendment, which in effect requries that physiotherapy be taught in our clinics, included a lead time of one year.

The Logan College Board of Trustees, at its June meeting, authorized Dr. Coggins to institute a physiotherapy course in the curriculum. Physiotherapy then can be taught. Physiotherapy then can be taught in the clinic. This will take most of the year to organize and phase in properly.[24]"

In 1976, certain members of the Palmer College of Chiropractic administration as well as some of the college's trustees proposed to include physical therapy teaching and practice in the curriculum. The combined efforts of Dr. David D. Palmer and myself were able to repel that action at the time. His position was the same as mine concerning the issue of physical therapy. Physical therapy is a profession, separate from chiropractic with separate qualifications for practice and licensure.

However, about one year later, shortly before Dr. David D. Palmer's death, a major change was made in the Palmer College of Chiropractic curriculum.

Yielding to the demands for accreditation, Palmer College of Chiropractic also included physical therapy as an elective in the curriculum of the college. It was stated 'to be used ancilliary to the spinal adjustments but not as therapies in and of themselves.'

However, the Educational Standards of the (CCE) Council on Chiropractic Education, March, 1978, page 37, carries this statement:

> "When the subject of physiotherapy is included in the curriculum, there shall be sufficient equipment for classroom and clinic purposes to insure a thorough knowledge in the effective use of all standard and acceptable physical therapeutic devices.[25]"

The Random House Dictionary of the English Language, Second Edition, Unabridged states these words regarding physical therapy:

> "Physical Therapy: The treatment or management of physical disability, malfunction, or pain, by exercise, massage, hydrotherapy, etc., without the use of medicines, surgery, or radiation.
> 2) the health profession that provides such care, physiotherapist."

And to emphasize again, physical therapy is a separate, accredited profession having its own standards in education and licensure.

Without question, the most revealing epitome relating to the mixer philosophy influence on chiropractic education is stated in these words by the President of a chiropractic college which is accredited by the (CCE) Council on Chiropractic Education.

> "While the C.C.E. has done much good for the profession, the A.C.A. influence and dominance of it has caused the traditional views of chiropractic to be nearly extinguished from the official academic mainstream of chiropractic, sweeping the

profession into an allopoathic frame of mind. Much like a frog in a pan of tepid water, which can be boiled without experiencing any pain, these institutions are being lulled into changes without ever being aware that traditional principles, the values upon which they were founded, are being boiled away.[26]''

Attorney Irving Kator, senior member of the firm of Kator, Scott and Heller, (Washington, D.C.) and formerly the Assistant Executive Director, U.S. Civil Service Commission has this to say about the mixer element of the chiropractic profession:

''*...if physical therapy is to be included in the curriculum for chiropractic training then such source of instruction should be approved by the American Physical Therapy Association and if medical practices are to be taught, then that course of instruction should be approved by the American Medical Association. Neither should be approved on the basis of a finding by the Council on Chiropractic Education which is not positioned either by virtue of its membership nor by its charter to certify to the quality of physical therapy instruction or to the quality of medical instruction, for that matter. As a result of the Council's actions, courses of instruction which are not properly accredited are being given to students and government funds are being expended for teaching which is not properly a part of chiropractic training and which in any case may be of only minimal value or of no value at all because whatever is taught has not been scrutinized by the proper approving bodies.*[27]''

The standards in education given by the American Physical Therapy Association in 1966, and again validated in 1976, state that qualified physical therapists should:

''Be a graduate of a physical therapy curriculum approved by the American Physical Therapy Association from 1928 to 1936; or by the Council on Medical Education and Hospitals of the American Medical Association from 1936 to 1960; or by the Council on Medical Education and Hospitals of the American Medical Association in collaboration with the American Physical Therapy Association since 1960; or a physical therapist trained outside the United States who shall be a graduate since 1928, from a physical therapy curriculum approved in the country in which the curriculum was located. The curriculum must be in a country in which there is a member organization of the World Confederation for Physical Therapy. Hold membership in a member-organization of the World Confederation for Physical Therapy. **Unless a doctor of chiropractic fulfills one of the standards described, we would consider that he is not prepared by his education for the practice of physical therapy.**[28]'' (Bold italic, mine).

My resignation from the Board of Trustees of Palmer College of Chiropractic followed the decision to include physical therapy in the curriculum of the college. I refused to be a party to the inclusion of physical therapy in the curriculum of Palmer College. The minutes of the Board of Trustees on August 17, 1977, show that my 'no' vote was so recorded, being the one and only vote against the establishment of a physical therapy clinic at Palmer College of Chiropractic.

My thoughts on this action were best summed up when I wrote to a member of the Board of Trustees of Palmer College of Chiropractic who had voted for the inclusion of physical therapy in the curriculum.

''In that one crucial vote, you and those who voted for

physical therapy, changed the direction of Palmer College of Chiropractic from a straight to a mixer institution." And the mixer smiled.

One can almost hear the words of Dr. David D. Palmer as he berated those who tried to include physical therapy in the Palmer College curriculum at the 1976 Board of Trustees meeting:

"*I'll close the school before I let it go mixing," he said as he pounded the table to emphasize his point! I turned to him and said: "You sound just like your good old dad, B.J." and he replied: "I can't help it, I am a Palmer. That's the Palmer in me."*

More than ninety years have passed since the principles and practice of chiropractic were first recognized and discovered. But much progress has been made in anchoring chiropractic within its true role. Favorable legal decisions give credence to the position that chiropractic is a separate school in the healing arts. Legislative bodies are becoming more and more aware of the chiropractor and the role chiropractic plays in the health services. A strong movement within chiropractic education is determined to set standards in education to qualify the graduate to practice a non-duplicated art. Dedicated, determined men and women who hold to the philosophy, science and art propounded by the Palmers press on. Chiropractic moves forward into the future keeping a freedom of choice in the healing arts for those in need of health care.

In August 1988 the Straight Chiropractic Academic Standards Association (SCASA) was officially recognized by the U.S. Office of Education as an accrediting agency for the chiropractic profession.

Educational recognition for straight chiropractic is one of the most significant, far reaching gains accomplished for professional advancement.

For chiropractic can now move forward within its own legitimate field of practice (additional details in the chapter on Education and Accredation).

References

1. The Science, Art, and Philosophy of Chiropractic, D. D. Palmer, 1910, pg. 18

2. Proceedings of the First National Congress on Chiropractic, April, 1967, pg. 35

3. The Science, Art, and Philosophy of Chiropractic, D. D. Palmer, 1910, pg. 11

4. The Science, Art, and Philosophy of Chiropractic, D. D. Palmer, 1910, pg. 14 & 15

5. The Science, Art, and Philosophy of Chiropractic, D. D. Palmer, 1910, pg. 101

6. The Science, Art, and Philosophy of Chiropractic, D. D. Palmer, 1910, pg. 105

7. The Science, Art, and Philosophy of Chiropractic, D. D. Palmer, 1910, pg. 17-18

8. The Science, Art, and Philosophy of Chiropractic, D. D. Palmer, 1910, pg. 18

9. The Science, Art, and Philosophy of Chiropractic, D. D. Palmer, 1910, pg. 18-19

10. The Chiropractor, D. D. Palmer. Published by Mrs. D. D. Palmer, 1914

11. The Science, Art, and Philosophy of Chiropractic, D. D. Palmer, 1910, pg. 8

12. Malpractice as Applied to Chiropractors, Arthur T. Holmes, 1924, pg. 188

13. Malpractice as Applied to Chiropractors, Arthur T. Holmes, 1924, pg. 188

14. The Evolution of Chiropractic, A. August Dye, 1938, pg. 91

15. Western States Chiropractic College, 1982-1983, Bicentennial Report

16. The Science, Art and Philosophy of Chiropractic, D. D. Palmer

17. The Great Divide, B. J. Palmer, D.C., 1961, Vol. XXXVIII, pg. 7

18. State of Michigan, Court of Appeals, March 21, 1983, Docket #61368, Attorney General on behalf of the People of the State of Michigan, Plaintiff, Appellee, vs James J. Beno, D.C., Defendant/Appellant

19. The Science, Art, and Philosophy of Chiropractic, D. D. Palmer, 1910, Preface

20. The President's Report, David D. Palmer, D.C., August 22, 1969.

21. The Superior Court of New Jersey, Appellate Division, A-1121-71

22. Accreditation Committee Meets, Contract for Binding Arbitration, November 10-11, 1973

23. Educational Standards for Chiropractic Colleges, March, 1978, Council on Chiropractic Education

References

24. World-Wide Report, Stockton, California, October, 1977, Vol. XIX, No. 10

25. Educational Standards for Chiropractic Colleges, March 1978, pg. 37, Council on Chiropractic Education

26. Dr. Sid E. Williams, President L. J. College, "The Leopard Doesn't Change Its Spots"

27. Attorney Irving Kator to Honorable Williiam Bennett, U.S. Secretary of Education, July 1985

28. Accreditation Status of American Physical Therapy Association Accredited Educational Program for Physical Therapist

CHAPTER IV

THE LAW AND CHIROPRACTIC

Today chiropractic is the largest non-medical profession in the healing arts. All fifty of the United States, the District of Columbia, Puerto Rico, Virgin Islands, the Canadian provinces with the exception of Newfoundland, as well as other countries have enacted legislation to license the practice of Chiropractic. Chiropractic is indeed a world-wide profession with an estimated 45,000 practitioners.

The history of legislative and legal recognition focuses clearly on the fact that D. D. Palmer's discovery in 1895, proved to be the basis for an entirely new and separate profession. Encompassed within his discovery is the understanding that an impulse energy circulation flows over or through the nervous system efferently from the brain to the body and afferently from the body to the brain. Interferences or interruptions to this flow of energy may occur if vertebrae become subluxated. Spinal adjustments restore the vertebrae to a normal position. In turn, the interference to the energy flow is released from the nervous system allowing for an innate health restoration.

"Chiropractic has its own particular practice of ascertaining the cause of disease and its own particular practice of correcting the cause allowing the innate force within the body to restore health. These attributes are the reason for it being a separate school in the healing arts.[1]*"*

And it was on these qualities as a separate, distinct

school in the healing arts that a basic, honest and fundamental legal grant was asked for and obtained in granting
licensure in the various jurisdictions. The chiropractic
profession fought for and won acceptance on the basis of
being a separate school in the healing arts. Licensure was
granted accordingly.

The struggle to gain licensure as a profession moved
into the legislative halls of the United States in 1910-11.
Legislative action was motivated to a large degree by the
constant and continued persecution and prosecution by
the medical profession. The charge 'practicing medicine
without a license' was the basis for their legal action and
harassment. Chiropractors were arrested. Many were
fined. Many served jail sentences.

The State of Kansas proved to be the decisive battle-
ground which rallied the forces in favor of chiropractic.
On March 20, 1913, the first legislative enactment to
license chiropractic was signed into law.

In her book, 50 Years of Chiropractic Recognized in
Kansas, written by Martha Mertz, D. C. are found these
words regarding the early chiropractors and their legislative battles to gain license. Dr. Mertz writes:

*"One must admire the courageous determination of these
pioneers, who like the religious reformers of past centuries, and
who risked imprisonment for their convictions in a better way of
faith.*

*Though this new science still had, and has even yet, many
refinements of technique to develop, it also has thrived on the
frequent failures which people experienced under medical care.*

*Many of those who took up chiropractic did so at an older
than usual age, having left other occupations due to their own
physical breakdown. Quite a few had been school teachers,
some lawyers or preachers, office workers and even druggists,*

*while some were farmers and housekeepers or wives of the men
who changed their life work and also studied with them.*

*Such mature years better guarantee an independence of
mind, willingness to withstand prosecution that others might
learn the truth of a new system of healing, which had already
been demonstrated in their own lives. They could stand alone
in their convictions, rather than conform to the crowd," con-
cludes Dr. Mertz.*[2]

Dr. B. J. Palmer was the rallying point around which
the effort to secure licensure was crystallized. He led the
action to defend those who were arrested for 'practicing
medicine without a license.' Dr. B. J. Palmer also led the
movement in securing licensure for chiropractic. He was
not only assisted by many chiropractors dedicated to the
cause, but many lay persons and members of other professions also helped. Among the most prominent was
Lieutenant Governor Tom Morris of Wisconsin. Working
closely with Dr. B. J. Palmer, Lieutenant Governor Tom
Morris was most instrumental in gaining legal decisions
proving chiropractic to be a separate practice and profession.

Dr. James Drain, a former President of Texas Chiropractic College, wrote in his bulletin, The Texas Digest,
1926, the following tribute to the Representative in the
Kansas State Legislature who spearheaded the legislative
action to license chiropractic in that state. This too sheds
light on the early struggle to obtain licensure. I quote
again from 50 Years of Chiropractic Recognized in Kansas
written by Martha Mertz, D.C.

Dr. James Drain had resided in Scott County, Kansas
before studying chiropractic. Following licensure, he also
practiced in Kansas for several years. He writes:

"The Chiropractic profession should remember H. A. Hines forever for what he has done for chiropractic. He was the first politician to pay any attention to chiropractic. He took up the fight in 1913, even though the odds were against him, and fought for and secured the passage of the FIRST Chiropractic law.

Eighty-six chiropractors supported him with telegrams and petitions. Mr. Hines went to the legislature from Scott County and argued that chiropractic was a science, not in any way related to Medicine, and it was entitled to a separate board of examiners, to be composed of Chiropractors. He fought the whole session, and the medical men opposed him bitterly. He told them that he was asking nothing of them nor any other science, that the passage of this act would not in any way affect any of the medical practice laws already on the statute books.[3]"

Mr. Jouett Shouse, a former Kansas Senator who fought for Chiropractic during the same session, made the following statement fifty years after the enactment of the legislation passed to license chiropractors in Kansas:

"It was my pleasure to assist in getting recognition in Kansas. It was merely a matter of justice as I viewed it."

Even though Kansas passed the first legislation to license chiropractors in 1913, because of difficulties in organizing the Board of Examiners, the first chiropractic license was not issued until May, 1915.

Meanwhile North Dakota enacted legislation in 1913 to license chiropractic and issued the **first** chiropractic license in the world in April, 1915.

Dr. B. J. Palmer gives this account of the early legal and legislative actions:

"During the past 42 years it has been necessary to observe closely and study carefully all events which did immediately, or might eventually concern the best interests of Chiropractic and Chiropractors. In the beginning we began our legislative activities with the informal assistance of Tom Morris (former Lieutenant Governor of Wisconsin), Attorney Fred Hartwell and other profound legal minds. They knew that definite and lasting security would only be assured by taking the honest, straight forward road to inform public opinion and support. A basic, honest, fundamental legal grant was asked, urged and received from the people through legislative representatives in most of the states. The issue was honestly presented and it was honestly argued that Chiropractic is a health science unto itself, separate and distinct from any other form or system of healing; that it has its own particular principle of ascertaining the cause of disease, and its own particular practice of correcting the cause and allowing Innate to restore health.[4]"

In the light of Dr. B. J. Palmer's statement, it is not difficult to understand the tremendous importance of the legal decision previously documented regarding the case of **Nelson vs. Harrington** 72 Wisconsin 591, 40 NW 228, (1888) and the legal requirements necessary to be a separate school in the healing arts. In various state legislatures, the conclusion reached in Nelson vs. Harrington for the requirements of a separate school were brought into focus as chiropractic pressed forward for recognition.

Dr. B. J. Palmer continues his statement in the Fountain Head News:

"In legal parlance, Chiropractic is a 'school of medicine' with its separate and distinct theory of 'Cause' and 'Remedy';

*the same as other 'schools of medicine', viz. Allopath, Homeo-
path, Osteopath, Christian Science, etc., which have been regulated by 'Practice Acts'. During these legislative battles to
secure fair and just legislative recognition of chiropractic, the
medical, osteopathic and legislator opponents always charged
'lack of good faith and honesty of intent and purpose'; they
stated that the 'license' to practice Chiropractic would not be
complied with honesty as a 'formal permission' from the proper
authorities to perform certain acts or carry on a certain business which without permission would be illegal." These opponents, medical and otherwise, charged that any separate and
distinct grant of 'license' to practice Chiropractic would be used
by many as an all-embrasive 'license' to do anything and everything they might decide in their own minds they wanted to
do.⁵''*

How true and correct were the oppostion's statements opposing licensure can and need only be determined by the practices which today are included in some
20 state's chiropractic practice acts. As stated in a previous chapter, these practices may range from practice
acts which hold chiropractic as a separate practice of spinal analysis and spinal adjusting to many others. Such
practices may include minor surgery, obstetrics, electrotherapy, hydrotherapy, colon irrigation, colon therapy,
physical therapy and many, many other practices of
other professions, each of which are not within the prov-
ince of chiropractic. The mixing segment of the chiropractic profession have, through their own means, been able
to convince legislators that they are learned in a broad
range of medical practices and physical therapy practices. The legislators of various states indeed have

believed their argument. It is however, most noteworthy in understanding that court decisions have constantly held chiropractic as a separate, distinct practice. Notwithstanding the practices of other professions which some chiropractic organizations, colleges and chiropractors have attempted to include as chiropractic, courts have been consistent in their interpretation in legal decisions.

The vast majority of states that have given license to chiropractic has been on the basis that chiropractic is a practice separate and apart from other professional practice. It was after their original, separate license was granted that the mixer chiropractic 'went to work' and in several states succeeded in convincing the legislative bodies that chiropractic had progressed into medical and physiotherapy practices. However, the fact remains that the original intent of the majority of chiropractic licensing grants was that legislation granted a separate, distinct practice for chiropractors. The example of 'chiropractic in Oregon' demonstrates the action of the mixer chiropractor.

Chiropractic licensure in the State of Oregon is a prime example of the results of this intra-struggle between the straight and mixer factions. The struggle is not unique to Oregon. Licensed as a separate, distinct profession in 1915, but fueled by the role of a chiropractic college in Portland, Oregon, which maintained the broad, mixer philosophy and practice, the mixer type chiropractic physician soon numerically vastly outnumbered the straight chiropractors. As a result, legislation licensing chiropractic as a separate, distinct practice has been amended as I view it from its original definition to the most mixed definition of any state in our union, even holding minor surgery within the chiropractic license.

The political power of the mixer chiropractic organization within the state forced the Board of Chiropractic Examiners to acquiesce in their favor in defining minor surgery practice. Education appeared definitely not to be the motivating factor.

The history of Chiropractic licensure in Oregon gives a clear history of the actions of those chiropractic physicians and chiropractors who fail to understand or accept chiropractic as a separate practice. The lure of being a chiropractic physician, practicing medical and physical therapy practices under color of a chiropractic license was stronger than straight chiropractic to those who, in my opinion, desired to be a medical doctor or physical therapist but found a way to gain a back door entrance to these practices without meeting education or licensure qualifications.

Chapter 325 Oregon Laws, 1915, carries the original definition of chiropractic.

> "Section B Chiropractic is defined as that system of adjusting the articulations of the bony framework of the human body, especially asymmetries of the vertebrae, for the purpose of removing the cause of disease by the correction of subluxations, thereby removing the pressure, impingement, or tension from the nerves having their passage between, through, or around the structures subluxated. The subluxation is corrected with the hands, using the bones of the body, more particularly the spinous and transverse processes of the vertebrae, as levers to which is applied a peculiar adjusting movement—the chiropractic thrust."

In clear, defining language chiropractic was adopted and became a new profession in the State of Oregon. The scope of practice was confined within the role of chiropractic as propounded by the Palmers. It duplicated no other profession and in turn was not duplicated by any other profession. A legal grant to practice a new and different practice from other professions was asked for and received from the legislative representatives of the people of Oregon. It was on this basis, as a legitimate, separate profession that licensure was granted. It is safe to say that if medical, physical therapy, surgery, optometry, dental, osteopathic or other practices were attempted to be included in the proposed legislation, licensure would not have been granted. Such clear defining language for chiropractic caused questions to be raised as to why, in later years, chiropractic statute language was amended to allow for practices foreign to chiropractic to be included in statute language. The mixer element of the profession, having failed to include their practices in the original licensing was relentless in its efforts to have medical and physical therapy practices as a part of chiropractic practice. Gaining a majority of licentiates, the move was made in 1927 to re-define the definition of chiropractic which had been held since first enacted in 1915.

Chapter 450 Oregon Laws 1927 re-defined:

>*"Chiropractic is defined as that system of adjusting with the hand or hands the articulations of the bony framework of the human body, and the employment and practice of physiotherapy, electrotherapy, and hydrotherapy, provided, no person practicing under this act shall write prescriptions for, or dispense drugs, practice optometry, or do major surgery; provided further, this act shall not be construed so as to interfere*

with or prevent the practice of, or use of massage, Swedish movement, physical culture, neuropathy, naturopathy, or other natural methods requiring the use of hand or hands.''

Somehow the mixer chiropractic physician type of practitioner was able to convince the legislators that chiropractic included these practices and that they were qualified to practice these other professional practices. It is important to note however, that to this day not one chiropractic college meets the standard for accreditation as adopted and propounded by the appropriate accrediting agencies for medical practice or physical therapy practice those being the American Medical Association and the American Physical Therapy Association respectively.

An amendment to the Oregon Chiropractic Statute in 1935, saw a further change. Glaring evidence indicates that political pressures by the mixer chiropractic organization other than educational advancements were ''calling the shots.''

Chapter 235 Oregon Laws 1935, under the heading 'Minor Surgery' reads:

''In order to clarify and define the scope of minor surgery as it is practiced by chiropractic physicians, the O.A.C.P., in convention July 1, 1936, at Portland adopted the following official definition and requested the State Board of Examiners to do likewise.

Minor Surgery ''That branch of surgery which consists of operative procedure by electrical or other methods, and which does not include the opening of the thoracic, abdominal or cranial cavities, or the amputation of limbs or extremities.''

''Notice is hereby given that the Board of Chiropractic Examiners, acquiescing in the request of the

association, has adopted the above stated definition
herewith advises all licensees of this board of its action
in this matter." (Bold italic mine)

Political pressures rather than educational excellence
again had its way.

In 1945, OCLA 54-301 defines chiropractic as follows:

"Chiropractic is defined as that system of adjusting with
the hand or hands the articulations of the bony framework of
the human body, and the employment and practice of physio-
therapy, electrotherapy and hydrotherapy provided that no
person practicing under this act shall write prescriptions for, or
dispense drugs, practice optometry, or naturopathy, or do
major surgery. (L-1915 ch 325, 8 OL 8618, L 1927. ch/
450. 3. P 670 OC 1930, 68, 915, L 1941, ch 62-1."

At the present time ORS 684.010 (2) is as follows:

(1) *"Board" means the State Board of Chiropractic*
    Examiners.

(2) *"Chiropractic" is defined as:*

    (a) *That system of adjusting with the hands the artic-*
    ulations of the bony framework of the human
    body, and the employment and practice of phys-
    iotherapy, electrotherapy, hydrotherapy, and
    minor surgery.

    (b) *The chiropractic diagnosis, treatment and preven-*
    tion of body dysfunction; correction, maintenance
    of the structural and functional integrity of the
    neuro-musculo-skeletal system and the effects
    thereof or interferences therewith by the utiliza-
    tion of all recognized and accepted chiropractic
    diagnostic procedures and the employment of all

rational therapeutic measures as taught in
approved chiropractic colleges.

(3) "Drugs" means all medicines and preparations and
all substances, except food, water and nutritional supplements taken orally, used or intended to be used for
the diagnosis, cure, treatment, mitigation or prevention of diseases or abnormalities of man, which are
recognized in the latest editions of the official United
States Pharmacopoeia, official Homeopathic Pharma-
copeia, official National Formulary, or any supple-
ment to any of them, or otherwise established as
drugs.

(4) "Minor surgery" means the use of electrical or other
methods for the surgical repair and care incident
thereto of superficial lacerations and abrasions,
benign superficial lesions, and the removal of foreign
bodies located in the superficial structures; and the
use of antiseptics and local anesthetics, in connection
therewith."

(Amended by 1953 c.541,2; 1975 c. 492, 1; 1987
c.726,1)

The actions in amending the Oregon Chiropractic
statute from one which originally carried the true intent
and purpose of chiropractic to one which was amended
to the point where it has practically lost the original
intent of the legislation is but one example of how the
chiropractic statutes in various states have allowed the
'mixer' philosophy to perpetuate itself.

In sharp contrast to the type of legislation allowing
chiropractors to invade and usurp medical and physical
therapy practices is that found in the State of Washington

which denies the right of other professions to practice chiropractic.

Section 7, added to Chapter 18.25 RCW, after defining chiropractic within the legitimate scope of practice are these words,

> "*Provided, however, that the term 'chiropractic' as defined in this act shall not prohibit a practitioner licensed under* RCW 18.71 *from performing accepted medical procedures,* **except such procedures shall not include the adjustment by hand of any articulations of the spine.**" (Bold italic, mine)

Chiropractic and the Law have gone through two distinct phases since 1895. During these years the profession has been established legally and legislatively. The latter stage, the legislative stage, is still being actively pursued and engaged in by the profession itself.

In the first stage of legal activity the majority of action took place in the court room. The medical profession constantly pressed the charge of 'practicing medicine without a license' on chiropractors engaged in practice. This was prior to licensure. The charge of 'practicing medicine without a license' led to court action. Decisions reached by the courts established legally that chiropractic did indeed meet the requirements of a separate school in the healing arts. The struggle to establish chiropractic legally was most important in the history of chiropractic. It provided the legal basis for chiropractic as a separate profession. For the courts have held that in order to be a separate school in the healing arts there must be rules and principles of practice which all of its members profess to follow. Chiropractic met those qualifications. It is a recognized school of healing with its own Art, Science and Philosophy, capable of being bounded and identified.

From this legal basis as a separate profession, chiropractic moved into the legislative halls of the various states to establish rights under chiropractic licensure. Such was essential, not only that chiropractic boards could be set up to examine chiropractors for the practice of chiropractic, but, also for another very real reason. Malpractice called for a profession to be judged by its peers. Having no license, meant that in case of malpractice, a chiropractor could be judged by medical standards. Chiropractic, of course, under these circumstances would not have existed long as a separate profession. Under such a condition, the standard of care would necessarily be the standard of care of the allopathic physician. Licensure was absolutely essential.

However, even under licensure, as the mixer invades the medical or physical therapy field of practice, a malpractice action allows for medical or physical therapy testimony as to the standard of care. A very real potential danger exists, if through such practices, the standard of care of a chiropractor is held to be the standard of care of the medical or physiotherapist practitioner. The very existence of chiropractic as a separate profession could well be threatened.

To clarify this point further, I quote from the Appellant's Brief in the malpractice case of Sheppard vs Firth, 215 OR 268, P. 2d 190 (1959), at pages 32, 33, 34, 35, and 36 as follows:

"*Respondent sought treatment by appellant, who she*

alleges, and it is agreed, was a duly licensed and practicing chiropractor: In treating respondent, appellant was not negligent because a member of the medical profession whose services are later secured, had no use for chiropractors and the chiropractic system and who would have treated respondent by his method rather than that followed by appellant as a chiropractor. A straight or regular chiropractor—and by that appellant means a chiropractor of the Palmer School and not a chiropractic physician who uses therapy and resorts to minor surgery—treats conditions of the spine, which was respondent's complaint, by the method of that school, namely, use of the neurocalometer and x-ray for analysis followed by adjustments to accomplish the desired relief. The medical profession follows a different system, that of diagnosis and traction or spinal fusion.

Appellant was entitled to have his treatment tested by the rules and principles of the school to which he belonged, that is the school of straight chiropractic, the Palmer System. This rule is followed throughout the United States in those states where the chiropractor is licensed as he is in Oregon. In malpractice cases the only expert who should be allowed to testify as to the propriety of the treatment complained of is one who belongs to the same branch of medicine or system to which the accused belongs. This rule was adopted in **Hilgedorf vs Bertschinger**, *(1930), 132 Or 641,285 P 819, and in* **Wemmett vs Mount**, *(1930) 143 Or 313, 292 P 93."*

Quoting further from Brief:

"There is no testimony or evidence of any kind in this case that appellant was outside of his system of chiropractic. His treatment fell within the scope only of a chiropractor who used that system, and neither John Frank Abele, MD, nor any

other member of the medical profession was qualified to express an opinion upon appellant's treatment. It is only in those cases where members of two professions use methods recognized by each, or, as is sometimes said, work in a common field that the one can testify concerning the work of the other. For instance, had the appellant resorted to surgery as do some chiropractic physicians, a medical doctor whose profession uses surgery would have been qualified to testify as to the propriety of the treatment. Or, for instance, had appellant used a diathermy machine, as chiropractic physicians sometimes do and as the medical profession does, then a member of the medical profession would have been competent to testify, as to the manner in which the machine was used. Or had appellant been giving x-ray treatments as chiropractic physicians sometimes do and as the medical profession sometimes does, a member of the medical profession would have been qualified to testify. Or had appellant attempted traction or fusion of the spine, in which field of treatment the medical profession works, a medical doctor could have testified as to the manner in which the treatment was given. Here appellant used a neurocalometer to locate the point of nerve pressure, an instrument of which the medical doctor Abele admittedly never heard and knew nothing.

*   *   *   *   *   *

Appellant took an x-ray of the vertebra to which the neurocalometer directed his attention as the seat of the respondent's trouble. There is no question here of the propriety of the x-ray.

Appellant is not charged with negligence in taking an x-ray so this gave no point of inquiry upon which the testimony of the medical doctor was competent.

Appellant made adjustments of the spine. The medical profession does not use adjustments of the spine as a method of treatment so the testimony of the medical doctor upon the matter of adjustments was not competent.[6]"

The decision was in favor of the defendant-appellant, P. B. Firth.

The State of Wisconsin in the Court of Appeals, District II, No. 86-0215, March 11, 1987, in Jerome Kerkman and Joyce Kerkman, Plaintiff—Cross Appellant vs Max A. Hintz and National Union Fire Insurance Company of Pittsburgh, Pennsylvania said, and I quote from a portion of the decision, pages 9 through 13, establishing a new standard of care for Chiropractors in Wisconsin:

"In light of these legislative pronouncements, we conclude that the **Keuchler** reasoning that "the practice of chiropractic is the practice of medicine" can no longer be viewed as an absolute statement of law in this state. The legislature has recognized that chiropractors and medical doctors are both members of the healing arts in that they are both ultimately concerned with the healing of the ills of their patients. Moreover, under the regulatory framework for chiropractors, chiropractic is at times a small subset of medicine, with the chiropractor able to use some, but not all, of the medical tools when analyzing and treating a patient. **See, e.g.,** Wis. Admin. code, Chir. 4.04 (chiropractor able to use x-rays to analyze patient's maladies). However, chiropractic only minimally intrudes into the medical field because chiropractors "are authorized to treat the sick only to the extent authorized by their chiropractic license." **Grayson**, 5 Wis. 2d at 207, 92 N. W. 2d at 274-75.

At most other times, the practice of chiropractic does not overlap into and is separate from the practice of medicine. Dr. John V. Whaley, D. C., a chiropractor licensed to practice in

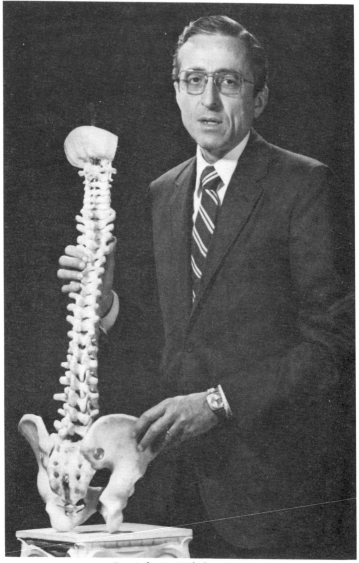

Dr. John V. Whaley, D.C.

Wisconsin and a graduate of the Palmer School, testified that a chiropractor does not treat or diagnose disease. Rather, a chiropractor analyzes a patient's spine and treats "subluxated" vertebra which may cause nerve interference. Dr. Whaley explained that "the chiropractic objective is to locate the subluxaton if it exists and then to adjust it back to its correct position with the objective of allowing the body better opportunity to restore itself." Dr. Whaley also noted that "the practice of medicine...the opposite (of the pracitce of chiropractic) because the medical doctor through the use of drugs and surgery and other (medical) techniques is concerned with...diagnosis and treating the diseased area." Dr. Whaley's testimoney is consistent with the legislative definitions of chiropractic.

Because we have concluded that the chiropractic standard of care set out in **Keuchler** is no longer valid, we are required to establish a new standard of care for Wisconsin chiropractors. In the medical area, we have held that the legal duty of a physician or a hospital is the reasonable exercise of that standard of skill and care which is maintained by the average practitioner or institution in the same class or professional calling, acting under the same or similar circumstances. **Johnson vs Misericordia Community Hosp.**, 97 Wis. 2d 521, 543-44, 294 N. W. 2d 501, 513 (Ct. App. 1980), **aff'd**, 99 Wis. 2d 708, 301 N. W. 2d 156 (1981). In addition, commentators have opined that the three main areas of chiropractic liability fall within the diagnosis, treatment and referral of patients. **See** Stutt, **Negligence of Drugless Healers-Chiroporactors**, Vol. 58, No. 7, Wis. Bar. Bull., 22 (July, 1985).

Based on these authorities, we conclude that chiropractors owe a duty to exercise reasonable care in the analysis and treatment of their patients which includes the duty to inform

2

them when non-medical treatment has become useless or harmful and medical treatment should be sought. **See Mostrom vs Pettibon,** 607 P 2d 864, 867 (Wash. Ct. App. 1980) _This standard of care requires a chiropractor to (1) recognize a medical problem as contrasted with a chiropractic problem; (2) refrain from further chiropractic treatment when a reasonable chiropractor should be aware that the patient's condition is not amendable to chiropractic treatment and the continuation of the treatment may aggravate the condition; and (3) refer the patient to a medical doctor when a medical mode of treatment is indicated._ **See** _id.:_ **Rosenberg,** _492 A. 2d at 378. In determining whether a chiropractor breaches these duties, he is held to the same standard of care as the reasonable chiropractor in the same or similar circumstances._ **See Mostrom,** 607 P. 2d at 867.

This standard of care is attractive because it measures a chiropractor's actions against other reasonable and ordinary chiropractors who are also restricted in their treatment by the four corners of the chiropractic license. **See Grayson,** 5 Wis. 2d at 207, 92 N.W. 2d at 274-75. _This standard of care also provides sufficient protection for the patient public because it ensures that a chiropractor will perform reasonably within the chiropractic field or face malpractice liability. Moreover, if a chiropractor performs outside the practice authorized by the chiropractic license into other areas of the healing arts, the chiropractor assumes the same standard of care mandated for practitioners in those areas and the corresponding potential for liability._ **See** _sec. 448.12, Stats._"

February 12, 1988, on appeal to the Supreme Court, State of Wisconsin, Kerkman vs Hintz, 138 Wisc. 2d, 131, 406 N.W. 2d 156 (Ct. Appl. 1987) the court **affirmed in**

part, and reversed in part and remanded. In the decision the Court said:

> "Because we conclude that a chiropractor should be held to a standard of care which requires the chiropractor to exercise the same degree of skill which is usually exercised by a reasonable chiropractor in the same or similar circumstance, we hold that the circuit court's instruction to the jury on the appropriate standard of care was erroneous. Accordingly, we affirm that part of the decision of the court of appeals which remanded the cause for a new trial in negligence. The question reversed and was remanded relative to damages."

The Court also held that a chiropractor does not have a duty to refer a patient who is not treatable through chiropractic means to a medical doctor. This is becaue such a determination could not be made without employing medical knowledge.

The division within the profession—the straight and the mixer has been a continuing struggle since the birth of the profession. That intra-struggle within the profession, between the straight chiropractic segment which desires to keep chiropractic as a separate, distinct practice, and, the mixer chiropractic physician whose desire is to mix medical, physical therapy and other practices with chiropractic under color of a chiropractic license, seems a never ending conflict.

In attempting to interpret or have an interpretation of a state statute so that the practice of physical therapy or medical practices might be included in the chiropractic statute, the mixing segment of the chiropractic profession have always met strong opposition by the straight segment of the chiropractic profession.

The first time the conflicting questions raised in this
issue relative to the **straight** versus **mixer** factions in chiropractic reached the California Superior Court was in
1933, as set forth in Dr. B. J. Palmer's book entitled The
Subluxation Specific—The Adjustment Specific, at pages
19-27 as follows:

> "*The People of the State of California, on the Relation of
> the Chiropractic League of California a voluntary Association,
> Plaintiff, and Cross-Complainant, vs. Roscoe C. Steele and
> Lois B. Steele, Defendants, vs. Glen Sipes and J. K. Christie,
> and Associated Chiropractors of California, a Voluntary Asso-
> ciation, Interveners and Cross-Defendants, Case No. 43645.*"

I will quote extensively from the decision because of
its importance:

> "*The issues, both of law and of fact, **are few and quite
> definite.** The Defendants have certificates issued to them to
> practice the healing art, under the **Chiropractic Act, and
> thereby licensed to practice chiropractic and not other-
> wise.** They hold no other license to practice any healing art in
> California. They are practicing, and are advertising and hold-
> ing themselves out to the public as practicing, certain modes of
> treating the sick or afflicted, termed opthalmology, nasal ther-
> apy, otology, intestinal flushing, pharyngology, laryngology
> genito-urinary therapy, proctology, irridiagnosis, scientific
> colon hygiene, sinusoidal current, ELECTRONICS,
> diathermy or artificial fever, d'arsonval auto condensation, cold
> quartz, ultra violet light, galvanic current and diet. These
> modalities, the defendants claim they are entitled to practice
> under their certificates issued them by the State, licensing them*

to "*practice chiropractic.*" *If this be so, the case of the State must fail; and hence* WE ARE *primarily concerned here with the proper construction to be* GIVEN THE ACT *under which their licenses are issued.*"

Further quoting from the legal opinion on page 22:

"*The defendants as heretofore stated, hold only certificates or licenses, issued under the Chiropractic Act; and the enabling part of that Act is contained in Section 7 thereof, reading as follows:*

17. Certificate to Practice. *One form of certificate shall be issued by the Board of Chiropractic Examiners; which said certificate shall be designated 'License to **Practice Chiropractic**' which license shall authorize the holder thereof,* **To Practice Chiropractic** *in the State of California as taught in Chiropractic schools and colleges; and also to use all necessary mechanical and hygienic and sanitary measures incident to the care of the body, but shall not authorize the practice of medicine, surgery, osteopathy dentistry, or optometry, nor the use of any drug or medicine now or hereafter included in materia medica.*" *On reading of this section, with respect to its application to the case at bar, two questions at once present themselves for solution before a proper conclusion herein can be reached.*

1. *What is meant by the use, in the statute, of the term* "*Chiropractic*"?

2. *How much additional license, if any, is conferred by the clause,* "*and also, to use all necessary mechanical, and hygienic and sanitary measure incident to the care of the body?*"

With regard to the first question:

"The word "Chiropractic" is a modern, fabricated word apparently from two Greek derivatives; and may be freely translated as "manipulation by hand." **It was applied to the system of healing, conceived and developed by Dr. Palmer, about forty years ago. He practiced and taught the system founding a school therefor, which was the original and central source of chiropractic theory and practice, and which is still functioning as the parent school of chiropractic."**

Further quoting at page 22:

Dr. Palmer defined Chiropractic as "...a system of adjusting the segments of the spinal column by hand only, for the correction of the cause of disease."

Another (Palmer) definition is as follows:

"Chiropractic is the science of palpating and adjusting the articulations of the human spinal column only." A third and more comprehensive definition which is found in Dorland's (Medical) Dictionary is "A system of adjustment consisting of palpation of the spinal column to ascertain vertebral subluxations followed by the adjustment of them by hand, in order to relieve pressure upon nerves at the intervertebral foramina, so that the nerve forces may flow freely from the brain to the rest of the body."

Continuing quotes from the legal decision find these statements on page 23:

"Without attempting to unduly prolong a discussion of the essential character of chiropractic theory, it may be stated, gen-

erally, that the science or art of chiropractic is found in these general propositions; that in the brain of the human animal is the point of control of an innate intelligence which sends its controlling forces by way of the spinal cord through the spinal column and then through the various nerve trunks emitting from the spinal cord and passing through the intervertebral foramina to nerve branches ramifying to all parts of the body, through the perfect functioning of which, health is maintained, but through interference with the transmission of those innate forces through or over the nerve, disease* is produced; that owing to the spinal column being the only segmented structure of bone through which these nerve trunks pass and the possibility of displacement of its segments changing the size and shape of the intervertebral foramina, subluxations occur and there offer interference with the transmission of innate forces directly or indirectly; that all disease* is thus traceable to impingements of nerve tissue in the spinal column. Chiropractic claims the knowledge of this all inclusive cause of disease* and the ability to adjust and correct these displacements of the segments of the spinal column, thereby removing interference with the transmission of innate forces. It claims that such adjustment does not add any material forces to the body, but allows the innate to restore to normal what it would have had, had there been no interference. In this manner, it is claimed, health is restored.

It will thus be observed that the theory, science or art of chiropractic is quite definitely circumscribed in its characters, scope and practice."

———

* *dis-ease*
* *corrected wording (all disease) dis-ease*
* *dis-ease*

It is always interesting to observe that when the court defines chiropractic or accepts a definition of chiropractic, it never wavers in the defining language. The original concept of the Palmers as to 'what is Chiropractic' is always the definition. In being circumscribed in its scope of practice, chiropractic remains separate from other healing professions. It contains the elements found in **Nelson vs Harrington** 72, Wisc 591, 40 NW 228, (1888). Further quoting from Dr. B. J. Palmer's book is this wording on page 23:

> "On the trial of this case, it appeared that there were two groups or schools of chiropractic which were generally referred to as "The Palmer Schools" and "The Mixing Schools"— these latter schools teaching the practice of the modalities, or some of them referred to in the pleadings here, and the practice of which it is sought to enjoin in this action. It is claimed on the part of the defendants that, because of the licenses or certificates of the defendants entitle them to "practice Chiropractic as taught in the Chiropractic Schools and Colleges" and such modalities are, in fact taught in these latter schools or colleges, that they are thereby licensed to practice such modalities. **With this contention the court is not in accord.** It is not alone the fact that the healing art which it is undertaken to practice is taught in such schools or colleges that entitles the licentiate to practice the same; but also that it is, **fundamentally or essentially, chiropractic.** The teaching of music may be carried on in a Chiropractic school, but that would not make music part of the art or science of Chiropractic. **There is no limitation upon what may be taught in such schools;** but

in order to render teaching of such schools the basis of the licentiate's practice, **such teaching must be of the art or science itself which must be chiropractic. By no stretch of the imagination, in the court's view can the practice of these various modalities complained of be brought within any reasonable construction or definition of chiropractic."**

The argument by the mixing segment of the profession "that the individual Doctor of Chiropractic has the privilege and the obligation to practice in accordance with his education received in a recognized college of Chiropractic," becomes moot when viewed in light of court language.

Again quoting from the Steele case referred to by Dr. B. J. Palmer at page 24:

"*If their use is justified at all by the defendants, it must be justified solely upon the theory that the practice of the same is permitted by the clause"...and, also, to use all necessary mechanical and hygienic and sanitary measures incident to the care of the body...*

It is the contention of the defendants that these various modalities may properly be practiced by one with a chiropractic certificate as being necessary mechanical and hygienic and sanitary measures incident to the care of the body. An examination of the character of these several modalities would seem to quite effectually answer this contention.

Diathermy, sinusoidal current, d'arsonval auto condensation are all therapies in which various forms of electrical currents are applied to the human body for various purposes—all of them possessing elements of grave danger when applied unskillfully—**and all of them being as far removed from the broadest possible concept of chiropractic.**

In the practice of modalities of proctology and so-called scientific colon hygiene, the practitioner inserts into the body, through the rectum, instruments and other substances up the descending colon through the transverse colon and down the ascending colon as far as the caecum, transversing practically the length and breadth of the interior of the lower abdomen. **By no stretch of the reason can it be said that this is a necessary hygienic or sanitary measure incident to the care of the body.**

Nor can the Court view the use of cold quartz or ultraviolet ray as a hygienic or sanitary measure or a mechanical measure incident to the care of the body.

Genito-urinary therapy includes treatment of all of the genitals and urinary parts of the body, and in these parts are the bladder, prostate gland and the kidneys; and the treatment of which involves the insertion into these parts of instruments, or other materials, and this, it is claimed, is a necessary mechanical hygienic or sanitary measure incident to the care of the body. **To state the proposition is at once to refute it.**

"The practice of opthalmology, or treatment of the eyes, nasal therapy, or treatment of the nose, otology, or treatment of the ears, pharyngology, or treatment of the pharynx, and laryngology, or treatment of the larynx, are all special therapies which are ordinarily committed even by those practicing under the all inclusive physician's and surgeon's certificate to specialists, and can, in the Court's opinion, **in no manner be brought within the clause of section 7 of the Chiropractic Act now under consideration; and are certainly far removed from any known definition of chiropractic."**

Dr. B. J. Palmer in his book set forth a copy of the Judgment at pages 26 and 27 as follows:

Endorsed and Filed: March 6, 1934

Henry A. Pfister, Clerk
By: E. T. McGhees, Deputy

JUDGMENT

This action came on regularly for trial on the 9th and 10th days of October, 1933, U. S. Webb, Esq., Attorney General Leon French, Esq., Deputy Attorney General and Frank V. Kinton, Esq., appeared as attorneys for plaintiff and cross-complaint; and Harry G. Henderson, Esq., Edward A. Stuart, Esq.,....and Homer J. Castellaw, Esq., appeared as attorneys for defendants, interveners and cross-defendants, whereupon evidence was adduced and the matter submitted to the Court for decision and judgment, from which the Court made and filed its findings of fact and conclusions of law:

NOW, THEREFORE, IT IS HEREBY ORDERED, ADJUDGED AND DECREED that the above named defendants Roscoe C. Steele and Lois B. Steele be and each of them are hereby permanently enjoined from practicing and/or attempting to practice and/or advertising and/or holding themselves, or each of themselves, out as practicing those certain systems of modes of treating the sick or afflicted in this State known respectively as irridiagnosis, scientific colon hygiene, sinusoidal current, electronics, diathermy or artificial fever, d'arsonval auto condensation, cold quartz ultra violet light, galvanic current and diet, and from thereby diagnosing, treating, operating for and/or prescribing for ailments, blemishes, deformities, diseases, disfigurements, disorders, injuries and/or other mental and physical condition or persons;

IT IS FURTHER ORDERED, ADJUDGED AND DECREED that the above named Glen J. Sipes, intervener and cross-defendant, be and he is hereby permanently enjoined from practicing and/or attempting to practice and/or advertising and/or holding himself out as practicing those certain systems or modes of treating the sick or afflicted in this State known respectively as opthalmology, nasal therapy, otology, intestinal flushing, pharyngology, laryngology, genito-urinary therapy, proctology and electrotherapy, and from thereby diagnosing, treating, operating for and/or prescribing for ailments, blemishes, deformities, disease, disfigurements, disorders, injuries and/or other mental and physical condition of persons, and from using in his practice the letters "E.T." as a suffix to his name.

IT IS FURTHER ORDERED, ADJUDGED AND DECREED that the above named J. K. Christie, intervener and cross-defendant, be and he is hereby permanently enjoined from practicing and/or attempting to practice and/or advertising and/or holding himself out as practicing those certain systems or modes of treating the sick or afflicted in this State known respectively as electrotherapy, radionics and radio therapy, and from thereby diagnosing, treating, operating for and/or prescribing for ailments, blemishes, deformities, disease, disfigurements, disorders, injuries and/or other mental and physical conditions of persons.

Let plaintiff have judgment for its costs.

WM. F. JAMES, Judge

Dated: March 6, 1934
Entered March 6, 1934, Book 32, Page 86."

The cliche 'history repeats itself' has never carried more truth than in 1983, almost fifty years after the California court's decision was made relative to the authentic scope of chiropractic practice. In the 97th Congress of the United States, HR 7097 and again in the 98th Congress, HR 31 was introduced on January 3, 1983. The proposed legislation sought to amend Title 10, United States Code, to include chiropractic care in the health care that may be provided to members and certain former members of the uniformed services and their dependents and to authorize chiropractors to be appointed as commissioned officers in the Armed Forces to provide such chiropractic care.

Opposing the passage was the Federation of Straight Chiropractic Organizations. This included those of us who know chiropractic to be a separate philosophy, science and art.

Does History repeat? Indeed it does.

Lines 21, 22, 23, 24, HR31 carries the purpose of this section: "(h) for purposes of this section, chiropractic functions include all diagnostic and therapeutic procedures taught in chiropractic colleges accredited by the Council on Chiropractic Education."

The Educational Standards of the Council on Chiropractic Education reads as follows:

"*The offerings should include the following disciplines: Human anatomy, biochemistry; physiology; microbiology; pathology; public health; physical, clinical and laboratory diagnosis; gynecology; obstetrics; pediatrics; geriatrics; dermatology; otolaryngology; roentgenology; psychology; dietetics; orthopedics; physical therapy; first aid and emergency proce-*

dures; spinal analysis; principles and practice of chiropractic; adjustive technique and other approporiate subjects."

In addition to these subjects, minor surgery, proctology, colonic irrigation, nutrition, counseling, orthopedic supports, orthotics (foot levelers) and casting are listed in one college of chiropractic accredited by the Council on Chiropractic Education.

Lab Services: Phlebotomy, EKG, six hour glucose tolerance tests, general chemistries and hematology are also listed.

Such practices could become a part of the chiropractic functions as stated in 'The Purpose of this Section' if HR 7097 was enacted into law.

In my opinion, public health demands that medical or physical therapy practices should not be practiced by the chiropractic physician nor the chiropractor unless and until the qualifications set forth by the respective recognized accrediting agencies for medical and physical therapy are met these to repeat for clarification once again are the American Medical Association and the American Physical Therapy Association respectively.

Those within the profession whose understanding of chiropractic provides an easy way to engage in medical practices and physical therapy practices without meeting the educational qualifications or licensure qualifications of practice attempted to militarily legitimize the mixer chiropractor and chiropractic physician through HR 7097. To this date, congress has seen the wisdom of not passing their proposed legislation. It would be a cruel hoax on the military and the American taxpayer if such legislation were ever enacted into law unless properly defined.

The language adopted by the U.S. Civil Service Commission for use in the Federal Employee Health Benefit Plans, defining chiropractic services to include spinal x-ray and spinal adjustments continues to be the guideline for federal legislation on chiropractic. This portal of entry as recognized by the federal government for chiropractic in health services serves notice that the only portal of entry into all areas of inclusion endeavors for our profession is confined within chiropractic's own unique principles and practice. Court decisions again stating the true role of chiropractic are having great influence on practice acts.

However, a major change had been taking place in legislative statute language since the Council on Chiropractic Education has been recognized as an accrediting agency for the chiropractic profession. The master plan of the mixer segment of the chiropractic profession called for a two-fold objective:

1. *Control of chiropractic education.*

2. *Control of state licensing practices. This called for either new statutory language holding that a graduate of a chiropractic college must be a graudate of a college accredited by the Council on Chiropractic Education or an amendment to the State Administrative Code with similar qualifying language. The clause, graduates from a college having standard equivalent to those of the Council on Chiropractic Education are eligible for licensure examination, was included to avoid legal charges of monopoly. However, by controlling the equivalency standards, the goal was the same. By 1978, over 40 states had enacted the requirement*

necessitating Council on Chiropractic Education qualifications or equivalency for licensure.[8]

This situation in which the straight segment of the profession was limited to less than 10 states in which graduates could practice led to court actions. Spearheaded by Sherman College of Straight Chiropractic, Pennsylvania College of Straight Chiropractic and the Federation of Straight Chiropractic Organization, numerous legal opinions upheld the fact that there actually were two separate philosophies in the chiropractic profession and one school of thought could not monopolize the right to practice.

A prime example is The New Jersey Decision.

The "mixing" element in the State of New Jersey attempted to prohibit 'straight' chiropractors from Sherman College of Straight Chiropractic to practice in that state. The State Licensing Board investigated. Their ruling allowed Sherman graduates to be able to take the exams for licensure.

After this ruling, representatives of the 'mixer' group filed suit against the licensing board demanding that Sherman College graduates be denied the privilege of sitting for exams. The case was decided in the State Court of Appeals with the Attorney General of the State of New Jersey defending the board's action. The straight school of thought was upheld in the decision.

The opinion written by Judge J. S. D. Morgan stated:

> "*Fundamental to CCE's rejection of Sherman College as an accredited school of chiropractic is the school's firm adherence to the 'straight' conception of chiropractic. The same reason underlies the negative recommendation of the chiropractors*

who passed on the school as members of the Board's (New Jersey Board) committee, both of whom seem to adhere to the ''mixing'' school of chiropractic.

Again the reason behind the College's lack of accreditation in several other states is its strict adherence to the tenets of the 'straight' school since many of those states require, as a condition to approval, accreditation by CCE which is 'mixing' oriented''...

Further quoting from the decision.

''When so analyzed, it becomes apparent that this appeal concerns primarily an attempt by one school of thought to deny entry into the chiropractic ranks to adherents of doctrine disapproved by them.''...

Judge J. A. D. Morgan further stated in his opinion:

''And as previously noted, lack of accreditation was based only upon Sherman College's adherence to the 'straight' rather than the 'mixing' conception of chiropractic practice, a distinction unmentioned in New Jersey law, and, in the expertise of the Board, of no significance to the qualifications of its graduates to sit for examination in New Jersey. We cannot substitute our opinion for the expert opinion of the Board.⁹''

Since the recognition of the Straight Chiropractic Academic Standards Association (SCASA) in 1988, as an accrediting agency by the U.S. Office of Education, the control of education and licensure previously held by the mixing segment of the profession has been nullified. Further clarification of such recognition is given in the chapter on Education and Accreditation.

A complication of legal opinions reprinted with the permission and my thanks to the West Publishing Company, St. Paul, Minnesota appears in the appendix* and was first published in the International Review of Chiropractic, Volume XX, Number 12, June, 1966, during my presidency of the International Chiropractors Association.

Quackery flourishes when one profession attempts to practice another's professional practice without adequate qualifications.

Just as quackery exists in my opinion when members of the chiropractic profession attempt to practice medical practices, physical therapy practices, or practices of other professions, without adequate qualifications so does quackery exist in the medical or physical therapy professions when members of those professions attempt to practice chiropractic without adequate qualifications. The chiropractic profession as well as other professions must 'police' itself to assure the consumer public of first-rate services in the health service fields.

By prior rights discovery and legally upheld position as a separate school in the healing arts, chiropractic must assume the responsibility of keeping its own house clean if it is to be a respected and accepted profession.

There is little question but that the profession must come together on its own scope of practice, uniting in a total effort to deliver its contribution to health services.

Until this time is reached, the immediate professional action necessitates divesting itself of any practices for which it fails to meet accreditation standards.

Painful as this may seem, in my opinion and in no other way can the profession of chiropractic reach its full

———

* Appendix B

potential in service.

The various and many practices foreign to chiropractic that are practiced under the name of chiropractic, have seriously hampered recognition and use of the profession. Why should people patronize those who would attempt to deliver services for which they are neither qualified or accredited? First class medical and physcial therapy services are already available from those who are properly trained and qualified.

Unless public acceptance is received and maintained the profession will not live and progress. Uniform legislative statutes confining the profession with its true role and scope of practice are absolutely essential. Confusion will then not exist as to the role of chiropractic. From coast to coast, border to border and around the world, one could be assured of quality chiropractic care. A total effort should be made to oust those from the profession who engage in practices foreign to chiropractic and for which they have failed to meet accreditation standards. Chiropractors must practice chiropractic. Will the profession do its own housecleaning or must others take on the task?

In clear concise language, Blacks Law Dictionary, 5th Edition, page 218, sums up the role of chiropractic:

> "*Chiropractic, chiropractics /kayrapraektak(s)/. The practice of "chiropractic" is a method of detecting and correcting by manual or mechanical means structural imbalance, distortion or subluxations in the human body to remove nerve interferences where such is the result of or related to distortion, misalignment or subluxations of or in the vertebral column.* **Chiropractic Ass'n of New York Inc. vs Hilleboe,** 16*

A. D. 2*d* 285.228 N. Y. S. 2*d* 358.360. A *system of therapeutic treatment, through adjusting of articulations of human body, particularly those of the spine.* **Walkenhorst vs Kesler,** 92 Utah 312.67 P. 2*d* 654-662.

The specific science that removes pressure on the nerves by the adjustment of the spinal vertebrae.[10]"

References

1. Malpractice as Applied to Chiropractors, Holmes, 1924

2. 50 Years of Chiropractic Recognized in Kansas, Martha Mertz, D. C. p 38-39

3. 50 Years of Chiropractic Recognized in Kansas, Martha Mertz, D. C. p 35

4. Fountainhead News, Dr. B. J. Palmer, Vol XXV, 1939

5. Fountainhead News, Dr. B. J. Palmer, Vol XXV, 1939

6. Sheppard vs Firth 215 OR 268,334 P 2d 190 (1959) at pages 32, 33, 34, 35 and 36

7. The State of Wisconsin in the Court of Appeals, District 1, No. 86-0215, March 11, 1987

8. A report on Chiropractic Politics and Education, Chiropractic Foundation of America, Inc. 1979

9. Superior Court of New Jersey. Appellate Division A-1121-71 In the matter of the application for approval by Sherman College of Straight Chiropractic Argued November 13, 1978, Decided January 5, 1979

10. Blacks Law Dictionary, 5th Edition, page 219

CHAPTER V

CHIROPRACTIC IN INSURANCE

Today, chiropractic is included in many of the programs at the federal level. These programs include, Medicare, Vocational Rehabilitation programs, Federal Workers' Compensation and several of the Federal Employee Health Benefit Plans.

At the state level, chiropractic is included in Medicaid and Workers' Compensation programs of each of the 50 states of the United States. Insurance equality legislation in over three quarters of the states require inclusion of chiropractic services in health and accident policies available in those states. Most major insurance companies include chiropractic in their policy language. Millions of people have access to chiropractic services in union, and health and welfare contracts. Many other countries also recognize and utilize chiropractic services in their health and welfare plans.

But this role of chiropractic in insurance was not gained without a struggle—a struggle for recognition and acceptance. And too, without the cooperation and dedication of many people who were determined that insurance should allow for a freedom of choice of health services, acceptance may well not have been accomplished.

''I have spent many years in behalf of the chiropractic profession on the local and national levels, seeking freedom of choice for the American worker who feels that chiropractic care is needed for his particular health problem'', so said the late

Rev. Joseph L. Donahue, C.S.V., Assistant to the President of the Chicago and Cook County Building and Construction Trades Council."

Rev. Donahue was one of many, determined that a freedom of choice in the healing arts was in the best interest of those seeking health services.[1]

But always hovering over the acceptance of chiropractic is the question—What really is the true role of chiropractic?

Charles L. Massie, a former President of the Government Employees Hospital Association (GEHA), one of the four largest Federal Employee Health Benefit Plans, stated his concern in these words:

> *"It is our opinion that chiropractic practice as licensed under the various state laws would be acceptable, providing that chiropractors confine their practice within the limitations and principles of their science, and further providing such practice does not infringe upon or duplicate any other healing arts licensed in that state such as medicine, surgery, physical therapy or any other related practice.[2]"*

Mr. Charles Massie was to become one of the most influential individuals in chiropractic inclusion and acceptance. He was most effectual in chiropractic inclusion in Medicare and the acceptance of chiropractic involving federal health plans.

It was my personal privilege to serve as Chairman of the Insurance Industrial Committee of the International Chiropractors Association, (ICA) and in this position to direct the action for chiropractic inclusion in insurance. With this background, I relate to you the factual history as to how a profession, discovered in 1895, deeply

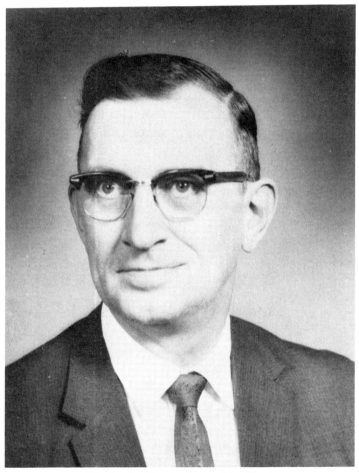

Charles L. Massie, former President,
Government Employees Hospital Association

divided in its philosophy and practice, even today—was accepted by insurance.

The late Dr. John Q. Thaxton, the second President of the International Chiropractors Association and Mr. Charles Massie were two of the most influential people responsible for securing chiropractic inclusion in the Medicare program. Dr. John Thaxton was a former New Mexico State Senator. He was a close friend of the late Honorable Clinton Anderson, United States Senator from New Mexico. Because of this trust, Senator Anderson introduced legislation for chiropractic inclusion in the Medicare program and was most influential in passage of this legislation.

Mr. Charles Massie appeared before numerous hearings of congressional committees relative to insurance inclusion. It was the experience with chiropractic in the Government Employees Hospital Association Plan that gave definition and factual statistics as to the worth of chiropractic. In turn this experience did much to convince Congress to include chiropractic in Medicare legislation. He relates the Plans experience in these words:

"Success of the GEHA the past 36 years both in rates of the plan and scope of benefits to our members has been based on availability to the membership in all areas of coverage in medical, dental and chiropractic services within the plans limitations in all three areas of service identity. Such contracts have kept the rate structure of the plan under control, and any deviation from this would not benefit our service to them, whether it be costs or scope or service. Any deviation from this would open Pandora's box to problems, misuse and less benefits to our members, or the American public. Doctors working

together in their capabilities will greater serve than attempting to duplicate those of other areas of help.[3]"

During the years of 1940-1950, the role of chiropractic in insurance was only sporadic in attempts to gain recognition.

No specific professional program had been enacted by the chiropractic profession either for the inclusion of chiropractic in the insurance contract, or, a program to confine chiropractic services to the legitimate scope of practice, or a peer review program as a part of a responsible profession.

Many chiropractors confined their work to the true role and intent of chiropractic submitting claims for spinal adjustments and the necessary work in spinal analysis.

But because of the inability to control the types of claims submitted for payment by many members of the chiropractic profession, the inability to reconcile grievances relative to claims, as well as the lack of cost control, insurance, in the main, avoided the use of chiropractic. Those chiropractors and chiropractic physicians who believed that a license to practice chiropractic gave them an unrestricted right to invade the field of practice of any profession or practice anything taught in a chiropractic college or licensed by a state as being chiropractic, submitted outrageous claims for payment. Claims were submitted to insurance for bloodless surgery, colonic irrigation, setting of fractures of broken fingers, setting dislocated shoulders, prescribing vitamins, use of Mayo cervical collars, steam baths, prescribing of drugs, ultra sound, physical therapy, hair analysis, medical treatments, psychotherapy and many other related medical and physical therapy practices. Little wonder it was that most insurance companies avoided chiropractic and refused to accept chiropractic claims.

Even today there are strong trends within some sections of the chiropractic profession to engage in 'sports medicine' practices. This practice involves injuries and treatment to the legs, knees, hips, arms, wrists and parts of the extremeties. Obviously, in my opinion, such practice is within the orthopedic medical field of practice and not chiropractic. If claims to insurance companies are submitted by members of the profession for this type of treatment, insurance may well reappraise the recognition of chiropractic services already attained.

Thus the continual same problem confronting the insurance industry in accepting and recognizing chiropractic services still remains. The lack of acceptance and recognition is still brought on by some members of the profession submitting medical and physical therapy claims for payment. This I feel even includes those states in which a chiropractic license allows for such practices. The lack of peer review committees within and representing the entire profession is a major factor in not adjudicating problem claims either as to scope of practice or costs submitted. Peer review is the mark of a responsible profession. Chiropractic must recognize this fact if confidence is to be maintained and established within the entire insurance industry demonstrating the efficacy of chiropractic.

I believe that the insurance industry must insist that recognition and reimbursement for claims be made only if the practices are taught in colleges accredited in those particular practices. Only then will the policy holder be assured of quality health services under the insuring contract. This too, should be the responsibility of the peer review committees.

In 1958, an in-depth study of chiropractic in insurance was undertaken by the International Chiropractic Asssociation. Dr. B. J. Palmer, the President of the International Chiropractic Association at that time gave the following guidelines for the program:

> "If the insurance industry can be so informed and educated that they will pay chiropractors only for chiropractic services, this action will do more than any other single thing to protect those insured from unscrupulous, fraudulent practices by chiropractors and it will do more than any action this Board can take to keep the profession within its rightful practice field."

The tone was set for an insurance and union industrial program that was destined to have a momentous, major impact on professional progress and acceptance for the chiropractic profession by the insurance industry.

To clarify chiropractic services and be of help in solving problems which might arise relative to chiropractic professional practices, travel by the members of the Insurance and Industrial Committee took us back and forth across this great country.

As an example, a conference with officials of a major Aeronautical and Aircraft Manufacturing Company in California, took place during one of our visits to California. This brought out some very significant facts.

A report by the late Dr. Frank Maurice gives this information prior to our conference:

> "In September, 1959, a four-man team consisting of two straight and two quasi-medics were invited to meet with the

vice-president and manager. After about 20 minutes of open discussion this executive placed upon his desk a stack of unpaid chiropractic claims no less than one foot high. He read about 50 of them to us. They were without exception outright medical bills running anywhere from $200 for an average low back pain condition to about $1,700 for 8 months of "treatments" for a sprained ankle on an 8-year-old boy. There were several bills of $3,500 to $4,500 for orthopedic services, traction, etc., over an 18 month period on a single case. To conclude the conference the Vice-president merely told the chiropractic group: 'We will not pay a single one of these bills until you people practice within the scope of the chiropractic law. We will give you 90 days to organize yourselves and to put a positive control on these violations.''

Dr. Maurice reports that the chiropractors did try to set up a control for abuses but were unable to accomplish the objective. Our International Chiropractors Association team was invited to meet with officials of the company at a later date. Our explanation of the role and scope of chiropractic practice as well as our World-Wide Insurance Review Committee was well received. We found the officials most interested in learning what the practice of chiropractic included. They were much interested in the fact that it did not duplicate or encroach into other professional practices.

Following our meeting, Dr. Frank Maurice reported that our efforts to explain chiropractic scope of practice, quality control by virtue of our review committee and the legal ramifications of our profession were successful. Chiropractic was again accepted.

The October, 1960 International Review of Chiropractic reveals the Statement of Purpose to improve insurance relations:

"The Board of Control of the International Chiroproactors Association has approved and directed that a World-Wide campaign be launched for the purpose of taking action that insurance policies include provisions for chiropractic care.[4]*"*

The October, 1961 issue of the International Review of Chiropractic carries these words, clarifying the intent of the program:

"The objective of the International Chiropractors Association program is to pull together all efforts presently being made, strengthen them and intensify their effectiveness. To do this, International Chiropractors Association has set in motion one of the most efficient task forces—a force of the best qualified public relations, industrial-insurance relations personnel—to soundly establish and represent the chiropractic profession with all major industrial and insurance programs as a major healing art and science.[5]*"*

The total commitment by International Chiropractors Association for chiropractic inclusion in insurance was a continuing effort by Dr. B. J. Palmer, Dr. John Q. Thaxton, and myself, as we served our respective terms as presidents of the organization.

The culmination of our actions at the federal level was realized in 1964-65. Chiropractic language was approved by the U.S. Civil Service Commission for use in the Federal Employee Health Benefit Plans.

The International Chiropractors Association program always identified chiropractic as a separate practice in

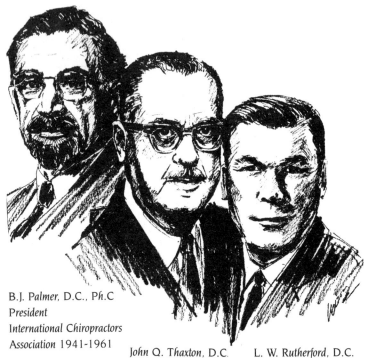

B.J. Palmer, D.C., Ph.C
President
International Chiropractors
Association 1941-1961

John Q. Thaxton, D.C.   L. W. Rutherford, D.C.
President   President
International Chiropractors International Chiropractors
Association 1961-1964   Association 1964-1971

the healing arts, being confined to spinal analysis and spinal adjustments. The language approved by the U.S. Civil Service Commission became the basis for defining language for chiropractic in the Medicare program.

Similar language appears as the basis of the AFL-CIO Executive policy for their membership. Under the insurance contract, chiropractic could demonstrate its worth. Acceptance of spinal adjustments in the health field moved forward.

Our conferences found the insurance industry confused in many instances as to what really was included in chiropractic services. Several company executives said outright that chiropractic was simply not recognized in their policy language. Others stated frankly that because of their inability to reconcile grievances and high charges made by some chiropractors, they tried to avoid chiropractic in their policies.

The great majority expressed gratitude to see the activation of the program by the International Chiropractors Association in 1960-61.

As before stated, the program included not only the introduction of the true scope of chiropractic but also a World-Wide Review Committee for claims review. Meetings were held with every major insurance company that indicated an interest. And the meetings with the insurance industry assured us that if our program met the objectives set forth in:

    a. Defining chiropractic in the contract as well as

    b. adequate peer review procedures, it could lead to the time that all insurance would recognize and utilize chiropractic.

This was our goal—inclusion of chiropractic within its own scope of practice in all insurance contracts.

Progress was being made. Insurance was beginning to have confidence. Chiropractors could and did perform a valued service to the policy holder as chiropractic was confined to its own practice.

When chiropractors submitted medical and physical therapy claims, insurance turned a deaf ear. Why should they pay for these services since the medical and physical therapy professions were already providing first-class quality service? The International Chiropractors Association took the position—pay chiropractors for chiropractic services only. We backed up our stand with a World-Wide Review Service. Chiropractic acceptance moved forward.

The massive program adopted and activated to include chiropractic in insurance in its true practice involved many chiropractors and friends of chiropractic.

Membership by the International Chiropractors Association in the International Association of Industrial Accident Boards and Commissions (IAIABC) organization played a key role in a better understanding and usage of chiropractic services for those in management as well as the insured. A continuing program was carried on. Today, every state recognizes chiropractic in their industrial accident coverage.

Membership in the National Conference of Health Welfare and Pension Plans gave further opportunity to explain and clarify the role of chiropractic. An understanding by many people at these conferences allowed for inclusion of chiropractic services in many levels of insurance heretofore not available.

The lesson which demonstrated itself consistently and positively as insurance accepted chiropractic services was clear. It is this—chiropractic must identify itself totally and unequivocally with the spine, and the practice of adjusting vertebral subluxations.

The Insurance-Industrial Relations segment of the program of the International Chiropractors Association set as a goal that of contacting and explaining chiropractic to each labor union that indicated an interest. And many learned of this truth of chiropractic for the first time. We advised the adoption of chiropractic language in the contract. With our Review Committee functioning, quality service and quality control could be maintained.

Mr. William P. Davis, having been a union member involved in union activities, was extremely helpful and effective in the program of chiropractic inclusion in the health and welfare union contract. Previously, Mr. Davis had served as Director of Training and Assistant to the Director of Industrial Relations for the National Tube Corporation, a U.S. Steel subsidiary in Pittsburgh, Pennsylvania. He also had been associated with Talon, Inc., the world's largest manufacturer of zipper products, serving as Superintendent of Production, Director of Training and Personnel Manager.

It was always our position that chiropractic services were separate and distinct—confined to spinal analysis and spinal adjustments. Chiropractic was a separate and distinct professional practice. It was on that basis, and that basis only, which we met with the unions and management. And it was on this basis, and this basis only, that chiropractic deserves to be a part of the health services included in the union contract or any other contract.

Said Mr. William P. Davis, regarding the union industrial program for chiropractic inclusions:

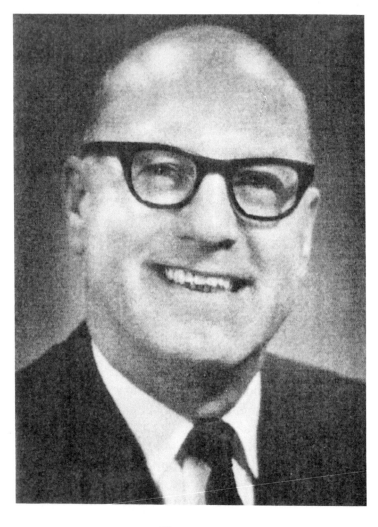

William P. Davis

"*Following our union contacts, especially those initially receptive to chiropractic inclusion, we made every effort to adequately inform them of the role of chiropractic and inform them of our International Chiropractors Association services especially as it related to our insurance review services on questionable claims. We made an all out effort to secure chiropractic inclusion in all major union contracts.*"

"*It should also be noted that payment for chiropractic care was secured in a great many contracts administered by Fund Administrators throughout America, particularly in the Midwest and Western States. In my opinion, the West Coast due to the influx of industry particularly aircraft, during World War II was far ahead of the rest of the country in establishing social and health and welfare programs, which were beneficial to employees.*"

"*The radical element of chiropractic, then and now, continues to undermine public confidence in the chiropractic profession.*

The 'mixer' element's lack of conformity and abuses contributed greatly to the reluctance of both Industry and Labor to accept chiropractic for its true worth and greatly retarded our programs for inclusion. Responsible management, union and insurance officials have stated that they would not endorse any health care service, which, by its nature and broad scope, would greatly increase costs, reduce quality of service and infringe upon the scope of practice of other ethical health care professionals.[6]"

Our program for inclusion of chiropractic was severely hampered by too many of the chiropractic profession crossing over into the fields of medicine, phsycial therapy and other professional practices. Such abuses

created suspicion and distrust among health care providers, insurance companies, management and labor
groups and the general public. They unwisely and unwit-
tingly gave the medical organizations all the ammunition
needed to combat chiropractic and to stifle its efforts to
gain its rightful recognition and status among health care
providers.

Continues Mr. William P. Davis:

> "No *industrial company or business can survive and/or
> succeed in today's competitive world without having a good
> workable 'Quality Control Program'.*
>
> *In view of the above facts, it was apparent that a program
> be developed which would provide the association and all its
> members with guide lines and standards which, if followed,
> would assure greater uniformity and raise the level of chiro-
> practic care to a more acceptable status among the other health
> care providers, insurance companies, industry and the public.*
>
> *Our efforts were well rewarded in the knowledge that
> many in the health and welfare contract would have a choice in
> health care when chiropractic was included. We feel confident
> that this, in many instances resulted in less time loss and a
> quicker return to work.*
>
> *The ground work which we laid could well point the way
> for inclusion of chiropractic in all union contracts. It would be
> our hope that this can become a reality.*[6]"

Since the insurance contract was rapidly and literally
becoming a 'way of life' in our society, the inclusion of
chiropractic services was essential if the profession was
to be able to demonstrate its worth to those insured.
Here again, the straight vs. the mixer scope of practice

posed a very significant question relative to acceptance. In a very real sense, the practical aspects of the mixer and straight practice became even more important than the philosophical differences within the profession. Inclusion or non-inclusion of chiropractic by insurance was at stake. The following question would be asked and was asked by many involved in insurance. "The insurance industry is already recognizing and paying for the first-class medical and physical therapy services, why then should insurance claims be paid to chiropractors for medical or physical therapy services?"

But the profession was to pay a heavy price for the mixer practices and philosophy which held that a practitioner was entitled to practice everything taught in a chiropractic college or included in state statute language as being chiropractic.

That price could have resulted in a complete elimination of chiropractic services as well as no recognition in all government approved insurance programs. Fortunately, this did not happen. As in so many instances, out of turmoil, comes clarity.

In 1965-1966, seven of the Federal Employee Health Benefit Plans had included chiropractic care in their programs. Chiropractic services were not defined. The words 'chiropractor' or 'chiropractic services' were inserted in Plan language.

Claims for chiropractic services submitted for payment included again, not only those for spinal analysis and spinal adjustments but also a vast cross-section of medical and physical therapy practices. Over charging also appeared as a common practice.

The World-Wide Insurance Review Committee of the

International Chiropractors Association was called upon for help in claim review and adjudication.

Our advice was consistent—pay chiropractic care for spinal analysis and spinal adjustments. But one claim submitted by a chiropractic physician was to bring a crisis to the profession relative to the acceptance or rejection of chiropractic in the Federal Employee Health Benefit Program.

Amid the confusion and conflict resulting from this chiropractic physician's attempt to collect monies for this particular claim would emerge an understanding and bring an end to the confusion as to 'what is chiropractic' in the Federal Employees Health Benefit Plans. The first defining language for chiropractic as approved by the U.S. Civil Service Commission for use in the Federal Employee Health Benefit Plans was destined to have a major far-reaching effect on all levels of chiropractic recognition and acceptance by the insurance industry.

The particular claim for chiropractic services submitted to the Rural Carrier Benefit Plan which resulted in the clarification of chiropractic services was as follows:

> "The patient was examined vaginally by palpation. Routine speculum examination revealed bleeding of the vagina but not the uterus. This was throughout the entire area.
>
> Routine physical examination revealed no prolapsis of the uterus, bulging, no herniation or accentuated increase in volume. There was no cystocele, no diverticulum, no cysts, no retrocele, no entrercele or other vaginal herniations. Routine lab examination failed to reveal any serious pathology. No sugar or albumin. Unable to demonstrate any trichomonads in the urine.

Physical examination revealed excessive tenderness in the area of the fallopian tubes and ovaries. No evidence of any defects in the surrounding areas of any consequence. However, the patient gave a history of suffering from extreme tenderness in the abdominal area for the past thirty years.

The patient was treated with positive galvanism, a fungicide, fluorescence with ultra-violet, and hot vaginal douches were also recommended. She was treated with ultra-sound over the affected area."

The claim was referred to the Insurance Review Committee of the International Chiropractors Association. Our advice was clear. Do not pay. This is not a chiropractic case. It is medical and physical therapy practice.

Because of non-payment, the chiropractic physician threatened legal action to collect for services. A real crisis arose as to whether or not chiropractic would be recognized at all by any of the Federal Employee Health Benefit Plans.

Finally a phone call from Mr. Andrew Ruddock, Director of the Bureau of Retirement, Insurance and Occupational Health, U.S. Civil Service Commission, asked me for an acceptable, true definition of chiropractic for use in the Federal Employee Health Benefit Plans.

I gave him the following language:

"Chiropractic is the philosophy, science and art concerned with the detection, location and adjustment of vertebral subluxations in the spinal column. Included in practice are the use of x-ray and other analytical instruments used to determine the presence or absence of nerve interference and vertebral subluxations. Spinal adjustments are done by hand."

This language was approved. It resulted in wording

being adopted by the U.S. Civil Service Commission for use in the Federal Employee Health Benefit Plans.

After the adoption of the intent of the language in the plan, the administrator of the Rural Carrier Benefit Plan made it known in these words:

> "It *appears that this case is now closed but for your information, this particular case has caused not only this Plan but other numerous plans operating under the Federal Employees Health Benefit Act to further define the scope of chiropractic as it will be recognized in the future. We have no desire to eliminate chiropractic completely from our contracts but it will be limited to spinal adjustments, including spinal x-rays to determine the presence or absence of vertebral subluxations or misalignments. This definition is presently being written into our contracts and no other chiropractic services will be recognized.*
>
> *It is unfortunate that we did not specify what chiropractic procedures would be covered in our contracts. Our definition of a doctor states he is a licensed physician, surgeon, osteopath, chiropractor or a dentist for purposes of services covered by the Plan. As a result of this weak definition, we will probably be obliged to make some payment on this claim.*
>
> *I do feel that it is my responsibility to advise other Federal Health Plans presently recognizing chiropractic services and also to turn over the complete file on this case to the U.S. Civil Service Commission for their future guidance in approving chiropractic services for health plans not presently recognizing these services.*[7]*"*

But the chiropractic physician mixer-type chiropractor consistently kept sending in claims based, as they said, on 'state law language'.

Finally on July 28, 1966, after valiantly attempting to

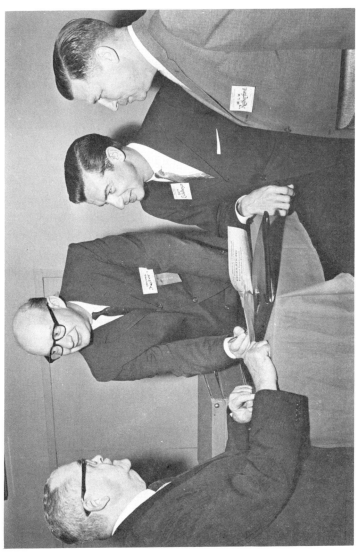

John Q. Thaxton, D.C., Attorney Irving Kator,
Mr. W. Scott Eichelberger, L.W. Rutherford, D.C.

hold the line on the mixer-chiropractor and project our profession within its proper confines, the late W. Scott Eichelberger, my good friend and Administrator of the Rural Carrier Benefit Plan informed me that effective January 1, 1967, chiropractic would be completely withdrawn from the Plan.

He went on to explain to me that the problems caused by complaints, excessive correspondence and the inability to reach an agreement with chiropractors and the chiropractic association representing mixerism or a broad scope of practice plus the inability to reach a satisfactory claim review procedure with the said association gave no alternative but to withdraw all chiropractic services. This is his statement:

> "It has been most difficult for us as the administrators to objectively decide the necessity for services rendered by some chiropractors and the reasonableness of the charges submitted, particularly in view of the fact that the two organizations representing the profession cannot agree on a common definition of chiropractic.
>
> The question as to whether or not chiropractic has a place in the healing arts is not in our minds, but the crucial question "What is chiropractic" is ever present. Until this question is answered, it is not likely that recognition will be extended by the majority of medical insurance policies, including the Federal Employees Plans and the laws covering Employees' Compensation and Medicare.
>
> We greatly appreciate the services rendered by your organization over the past six years and wish you success in your goal to obtain an acceptable 'scope of practice' for the chiropractic profession.[8]"

A sordid chapter in the history of the chiropractic profession was written at the Federal level by those who held to the philosophy that anything taught in a chiropractic college or enacted in state statute language was included in chiropractic practice.

Plan administrators know better than many in the profession the role of chiropractic. Four of the Federal Employee Health Benefit Plans removed chiropractic services from Plan language.

Conflicts clarify. The controversy resulted in a clarification. Language properly defining chiropractic was approved by the U.S. Civil Service Commission for use in the Federal Emloyee Health Benefit Plans. This would lay the groundwork for acceptance and definition in Medicare and other far-reaching insurance programs.

Recognition of chiropractic services at the federal level were influenced greatly by the defining of chiropractic services for the Federal Employee Health Benefit Plans. The Federal Employees Compensation Act defined legislation relative to chiropractic services. Mr. Charles Massie gave pertinent testimony on the issue:

> ''*Chiropractic services shall be reimbursed only for spinal adjustments by hand and spinal x-rays. It is our opinion that the Federal Government has much to gain in recognition of chiropractic care in the Federal Employees Compensation Act through the availability to a source of healing arts that will enable an employee to return to duty at an early a date as possible following a work-related injury.*
>
> *May we respectfully submit that your deliberations be made on specific controls on scope of practice and not on scope*

of license since there is a wide variance between state laws and regulations covering chiropractic.

It is my understanding that the International Chiropractors Association accepts and approves the terminology used in definitive language of chiropractic by our Plan, and I sincerely trust that this information will serve some purpose in your deliberations. We believe that the Federal employee should have the right to select from the field of healing art services most applicable to his earliest and complete recovery.⁹''

Legislation was enacted into law including chiropractic as defined.

Another who was most helpful and who must be mentioned in any legislation enacted at the federal level for chiropractic inclusion is Brigadier General Joseph P. Adams. General Adams served the International Chiropractors Association as Counsel and representative in the nation's capitol for many years.

One further statement on Mr. Massie's position on the role in chiropractic is found in his letter written to me as President of the International Chiropractors Association, August 12, 1966, wherein he states:

''It seems strange to me as a plan administrator that many chiropractors cannot and do not confine their activities to their special area of practice, namely spinal analysis and spinal adjustments. Why must they engage in the practice of diagnosis, medical treatments, medical practices, and the work of the physiotherapist. We are already paying for these services under the medical provisions of our program. Chiropractors have a separate service to render to be recognized as a separate profession, and only through such do they warrant inclusion.

*To this date we have never had a claim submitted by a medical doctor or physiotherapist for spinal adjusting. Why is it that some members of your profession feel that they must indulge in other professional practices when they do have a **real specific service** to render in their own field. Is it possible they have little or no faith in chiropractic; our experience has shown a real service rendered by your profession in spinal analysis and spinal adjusting, and only in this do we have faith in chiropractic.[10]*

Chiropractic will need to do more than ape the medical practitioner or the physical therapist to be accepted into the mainstream of insurance. The chiropractic profession must demonstrate the worth and value of spinal adjustments in health restoration and maintenance. A total concerted effort by the chiropractic profession based entirely on the principles and practice of chiropractic inherent within spinal adjusting would not only be a tremendous service to mankind but could firmly anchor chiropractic and light its potential for helping sick people get well.

Statements such as the following gave much encouragement to our program, said Floyd E. Smith, President, International Association of Machinists:

"I want my Union Members to have the right to choose— it is our moral responsibility to provide a better life for the generation we are now raising, and because I believe that union members should have the right to select their health care and because the members of International Chiropractors Association are interested in providing that health care, I want the International Chiroporactors Association and chiropractic to be as strong as possible so my members can benefit.[11]"

There are few areas of human endeavor that touch and influence so many lives as the insurance contract. John Grogan, President, Industrial Union of Marine and Shipbuilders stated:

> "We in the American Labor movement know that your great honored profession is one that the people of our country need.[12]"

The late Patrick Gorman, Amalgamated Meat Cutters and Butcher Workman was very instrumental in affecting inclusion of chiropractic within its proper role in the Union contract.

The Butcher Workman, the magazine of the Amalgamated Meat Cutters and Butcher Workman of North Amercia carried a news story entitled "Unions Include Chiropractic Services Benefits in Contracts."

> "Inclusion of chiropractic benefits in contracts, usually at no additional cost, provides members greater freedom of choice between the various types of doctors and prevents the necessity of members having to pay for chiropractic services when such services are needed. Coverage is included for spinal adjustments and spinal instrumentation, including x-ray.
>
> The trend toward the general inclusion of chiropractic within the union movement is partially the result of close liaison work between the International Chiropractors Association and the union movement to develop improved understanding of the chiropractic healing art and its steady and substantial growth in the country.
>
> It is also the result of the growing awareness of the efficiency of chiropractic particularly with back injuries often caused by accidents. One out of every 10 lost-time injuries is

the result of back strain. Dr. Rutherford pointed out that both on and off the job accidents are making back injury as common as the common cold."

These people are representative of friends in union and management. The list is long. My thanks to each for participating in keeping and projecting a freedom of choice for chiropractic services for those in need. Quality control, cost control and chiropractic confined within its own principles and practice were the issues on which our program for inclusion were based as we met with management and representatives of the vast majority of labor unions.

The AFL-CIO adopted this position on Coverage of Chiropractic Services in Government Programs, May 19, 1976.

"We do not believe that chiropractors should attempt to perform the functions of physicians or surgeons for which they are unqualified. Where they attempt to perform such functions, we oppose such practice.

Until adequate research indicates to the contrary, chiropractic services should be restricted to treatment of subluxations of the spine, the particular condition that falls within the competency of chiropractic, plus related and necessary x-rays, physical examinations, and diagnostic service to assure that chiropractic treatment is in order. In recently passed social security legislation, Congress included chiropractic services under Medicare and Medicaid, but only with respect to treatment by means of manual manipulation of the spine and only with respect to subluxation of the spine demonstrated by x-ray.

We urge that if chiropractic services are included in any other public programs, such coverage be subject to the same

*restrictions, plus related and necessary x-rays, physical exami-
nations and diagnostic services to assure that chiropractic is in
order.*[13]"

The program for chiropractic inclusion in insurance
was a massive ongoing effort by the International Chiropractors Association. Quality control within the principles
and practice of chiropractic was the guideline. But as
always, and even today, the scope of chiropractic practice
continues to plague the profession.

To overcome this long-standing question of definition
and scope of practice; to adopt a common language for
the insurance report; to establish world-wide peer review
committees; to assure the insurance industry that all chiropractors will confine their practice to chiropractic's
rightful role—these are the challenges for the chiropractic
profession. For chiropractic in the insurance contract can
prove its worth, both to the insurer and the insured in
health restoration and maintenance.

References

1. Rev. Joseph L. Donahue, C.S.V., 1980 to General President United Rubber Workers.

2. Charles L. Massie, letter to L. W. Rutherford, D.C.

3. Charles L. Massie, letter to L. W. Rutherford, D.C.

4. International Review of Chiropractic, October, 1960.

5. International Review of Chiropractic, October, 1961.

6. Statement of William P. Davis

7. W. Scott Eichelberger to Edward J. Lyons of ICA.

8. W. Scott Eichelberger to L. W. Rutherford.

9. Charles L. Massie to Honorable Lee Metcalf, Chairman United States Committee on Labor and Public Welfare. Special Committee Federal Employee Compensation, July 2, 1964.

10. Charles L. Massie, to L. W. Rutherford, D.C., August 12, 1966.

11. International Review of Chiropractic, 1964, Floyd E. Smith, General Vice-President (later President) International Association of Machinists.

12. International Review of Chiropractic, May, 1963. John Grogan, President Industrial Union of Marine and Shipbuilders, AFL-CIO.

13. Statement - AFL-CIO, Executive Council on Coverage of Chiropractic Services in Government Programs, May 19, 1976, Washington, D.C.

CHAPTER VI

EDUCATION AND ACCREDITATION

Accreditation brings new responsibility to chiropractic and the chiropractic profession. As the accreditation of chiropractic becomes a reality, chiropractic must respect the standards and criteria of each and every accrediting agency recognized by the U.S. Office of Education if it is to be recognized as an accrediting agency for the chiropractic profession.

No longer can chiropractic qualify for another profession's practice merely by broadening of a legislative statute including other professional practices within statute language as chiropractic. Neither does chiropractic qualify for another professional practice merely by the subject matter being taught in a chiropractic college. Accreditation standards for those practices must **be met.** Public health demands this protection.

No longer can the chiropractic profession remain an undefined profession in scope of practice and definition. Accreditation adds a new dimension to chiropractic understanding and meaning. Accreditation saddles the profession with the same responsibilities as it does the other professions in seeing to it that adequate legitimate standards are met and maintained. In chiropractic this is the responsibility in meeting standards of excellence in chiropractic principle and practice so that the seeker of chiropractic care will be assured of quality service.

Among its goals, accreditation assures the educational community as well as the public that an institution meets certain standards in quality education. This would also extend to all other areas in which it might have an involvement such as private or public agencies.

Accreditation is also an eligibility requirement which must be met to determine if an educational institution is eligible to participate in government programs involving federal funds. And with these facts as a yardstick, the chiropractic profession must re-assess its total position on the health scene.

An important question is raised in this respect. Can dual or double standards for the practice of the same professions be acceptable for accreditation and recognition by the Office of Education? To repeat, not one chiropractic college meets the standards for the practice of physical therapy as adopted by the American Physical Therapy Association; the accrediting organization for this profession. Not one chiropractic college meets the accrediting standards for the practice of medical practices as adopted by the American Medical Association, the accrediting organization for this profession.

A chiropractic accrediting agency is not, in my opinion, qualified to accredit educational standards for these professions. And yet, the plain simple fact is that the Council on Chiropractic Education (CCE) is functioning as an accrediting body, recognized by the U.S. Office of Education, and is accrediting chiropractic colleges teaching physical therapy and medical practices.

Surely the public is entitled to proper and adequate protection from the unqualified practitioner. More especially is this a matter of public concern since Federal funds are being allocated to provide for medical and physical therapy education in chiropractic colleges accredited by the Council on Chiropractic Education.

In the interest of public health and safety, I feel that questions must be asked and most certainly deserve an answer since dual accreditation of medical and physical therapy practices is a paramount issue and question.

Is the Council on Chiropractic Education a legitimate accrediting agency for medical and/or physical therapy practices?

Are the educational standards long recognized by the accrediting agencies for medical and/or physical therapy practices being met or equalled by accredited chiropractic colleges?

In my opinion, public health and safety demands the same educational standards should prevail relative to medical practices in a chiropractic college teaching medical practices as are found in a medical college.

Likewise, in my opinion, the same educational standards should prevail relative to physical therapy practices in a chiropractic college teaching physical therapy practices as are found in a physical therapy institution teaching similar practices.

For as I understand it, the U.S. Office of Education holds to the policy that it is not the profession which is being accredited, rather it is education which is being accredited. Accordingly, the allocations and use of federal and/or state funds should be measured by the yardstick of the adequacy and quality of education. An investigation should give the facts. Adequacy in meeting the test of quality education could only be a compliment to the educational process. By the same yardstick, inadequacy in education should not be tolerated but rather should be eliminated.

Unless the quality of education meets the educational

accreditation standards, public monies should not become a part of the program for support.

In the public interest, a determination must be made as to whether or not the Council on Chiropractic Education (CCE) is a "reliable authority on the quality of training in chiropractic colleges" specifically and directly directed as to the teaching, practice, and accreditation of physical therapy and its practices being taught in chiropractic colleges.

In the public interest, a determination must be made as to whether or not the Council on Chiropractic (CCE) is a "reliable authority on the quality of training in chiropractic colleges" specifically and directly directed as to the teaching, practice, and accredition of all medical practices being taught in chiropractic colleges.

For as long as doubt prevails regarding these practices, the question remains unanswered.

The role of chiropractic teaching must be clarified, for surely among its goals, accreditation assures the public as well as the educational community that an institution meets certain standards in quality education.

A chiropractic education should equip the graduate to practice chiropractic. In the foregoing chapters I have delineated the scope of chiropractic practice along with the attempts by some to gain rights to other professional practice rights under the guise of chiropractic.

Sherman College of Straight Chiropractic carried this wording in the Announcement section of the college bulletin setting a theme for education.

"Since the best potter must have good material with which to fashion his product, we all look for students that have the

capacity and attributes necessary for becoming outstanding Doctors of Chiropractic. Such students must first possess a love for people and a deep respect for life itself. They also must have inquisitive minds and find beauty in truth that cannot be compromised. As Doctors of Chiropractic our graduates will be challenged, not only by the uniqueness of each patient's spinal problem but also by presenting to humanity a new idea— knowing that humanity inherently resists new ideas.'''

The field of chiropractic offers one of the most, if not the most, tremendously challenging endeavors in the healing arts.

The potential is practically unlimited in service. When one considers that each individual has a spinal column and that only the chiropractor concentrates on work which releases interferences in the nervous sytem if spinal bones become subluxated, it is easily understood that the chiropractor plays a most important role in helping to solve humanity's problems relating to the spine.

That challenge to help humanity through spinal adjustments has carried chiropractic around the world. As the potential inherent within the idea conceived by D. D. Palmer in 1895 becomes fully understood, the colleges of chiropractic will be hard pressed to meet the demand.

It is my firm belief that the graduate must have ample exposure to today's educational opportunities and background to be able to assume the true role and responsibility demanded of the Doctor of Chiropractic.

I will not in this work attempt to detail the subject matter required in a chiropractic college curriculum.

Suffice to say that education should be directed to a

broad knowledge of the body in general and the spine and nervous system and the practice of chiropractic in particular.

Practices of other professions such as a medical, physical therapy, optometry, and orthopedics practices should in no way be a part of a chiropractic curriculum. These are totally unjustified in a chiropractic college teachings for the very basic facts that these practices fail to meet accreditation standards in a chiropractic college. In no way can they be construed to be the practice of chiropractic. Court decisions over the years have made this abundantly clear.

The art of locating and of adjusting subluxated vertebrae should consume a major portion of chiropractic teaching. The study of the impulse energy flow over the nervous system itself should be a major central theme in the curriculum. In this electronic age the chiropractic profession should be in the forefront in the research and development of instruments to record the impulse energy flow over and through the nervous system when vertebra are subluxated and when adjusted. Instruments such as I have already indicated which were used in the late B. J. Palmer Chiropractic Research Clinic to record temperature differentials such as the neurocalograph and to record the energy impulse flow over the nervous system such as the electroencephaloneuromentimpograph as well as precision x-rays of the spine, all and each of these should assume a major role in chiropractic education.

The next few years may witness wider use of instruments used in spinal adjusting as more exact means and methods are devised to adjust the vertebral subluxation.

However, I would suggest that it would be a long time before these instruments replace the hands for use in spinal adjusting.

Nevertheless as proof is demonstrated regarding the ability to correctly adjust the subluxation with instruments, instrumentation methods may gradually replace hand adjusting of the spine.

If the chiropractor is to survive and progress in the years ahead, it will be because of the ability to locate and adjust the vertebral subluxation. This worth and value of chiropractic in health maintenance and restoration will then take its place in the mainstream of the healing arts as a separate practice. Education should be geared to this purpose.

Chiropractic accreditation must hold the educational requirements to educate the chiropractor within the separate, distinct school in the healing arts embodied in the exclusive chiropractic principle and practice.

If education is the molder of minds as is sometimes said it is, it is indeed capable of being the molder of professions.

The latest in the saga of the mixer education move into the mainstream of medical practice is proposed in legislation in the 84th General Assembly, State of Illinois 1985-1986, to amend the medical practice act. A chiropractor is considered a physician under Illinois law and is now considered to be one who 'treats human ailments without the use of drugs, medicines or operative surgery.' The proposed legislation reads as follows:

"Section 15. Any physician licensed under this Act to treat human ailments without the use of prescriptive drugs and

operative surgery shall be permitted to take the examination provided for under Section 13 of this Act and shall receive a license to practice medicine in all of its branches if he or she shall successfully pass such examination, upon proof of having successfully completed in a medical college, osteopathic college or chiropractic college reputable and in good standing in the judgment of the Department, courses of instruction in materia medica, therapeutics, surgery, obstetrics, and theory and practice deemed by the Department to be equal to the courses of instruction required in those subjects for admission to the examination for a license to practice medicine in all of its branches, together with proof of having completed (a) the two years' course of instruction in a college of liberal arts, or its equivalent, required under this Act, and (b) a course of post-graduate clinical training of not less than 24 months as approved by the Department.[2]"

Section 15 became a part of the State of Illinois Medical Practice of 1987, which was enacted into law.

While this equally may belong in the discussion on legislation, nevertheless the proposed education of the chiropractor from a separate non-duplicated practice to that of medical practitioner is most significant in this legislation. Could this possibly be the beginning pattern of the absorption by allopathic medicine of the chiropractic idea and profession?

It is my considered opinion that eventually if this profession is to reach full acceptance as a profession identified as a separate school in the healing arts, the colleges must become integrated into the higher educational system of each jurisdiction.

But safe to say, until chiropractic colleges divest

themselves of any teaching leading to practices of professions other than chiropractic, the college educational program of chiropractic will be looked upon with suspicion and disrespect by higher education.

Recognizing the facts that an accrediting agency must be organized to adequately represent chiropractic within its true and legal parameters, in 1979, The Committee on Accreditation of the Straight Chiropractic Academic Standards Association (COA) was founded.[3]

In the Historical Statement is this wording:

> "In the latter part of 1977 it became obvious to many that a chasm had developed within the chiropractic profession to the degree that a reunification of the profession was impossible. Observers were led to conclude that not only was there an existing chasm; indeed there existed two separate professions within one profession. It was widely observed that the separation was not fundamentally political; it was philosophical and essential.
>
> The pivotal point in the division of the two branches centered around the direction of chiropractic objectives. One branch fully endorsed the position that the objective of chiropractic was the diagnosis and treatment of disease. The other branch was just as firmly committed to (a) fighting the objective of "diagnosis and treatment"; and (b) espousing the sole objective of "removing interferences" to the body's own propensity to heal itself."

It can readily be seen that the objectives of each segment of the profession were so far removed that there actually were two professional practices under the banner of chiropractic.

Further quoting from the same source, may give a

better understanding of how and why a new accrediting
agency was formed:

"Each branch had developed separately and uniquely.
Existing institutions and organizations responded to each
branch based primarily on their own interpretations of chiropractic objectives. Likewise, new organizations were created to
fill vacuums that existed by the separate development of the two
chiropractic professions.

Within this context, a major concern developed as to the
need for the creation of an accrediting agency to evaluate the
chiropractic colleges which espoused "straight" chiropractic
objectives.

Concern was expressed in meetings, addresses, publica-
tions and correspondence. The concern was so pervasive that an
ad hoc committee was formed to lead in the development of a
new accrediting agency to serve the public and the profession
by evaluating straight chiropractic colleges.

Late 1977. In late 1977, an **ad hoc** committee was
formed, and out of that committee came a strong momentum to
move ahead with the formal creation of a straight chiropractic
accrediting association. Straight chiropractic objectives were
discussed at length, and a growing consensus evolved as to the
concepts of objectives, organization, programs and time frame.

A name was selected: The Straight Chiropractic Academic
Standards Association. The effort became commonly referred to
as S.C.A.S.A.

After innumerable meetings and much study of the purposes and programs, on September, 1979, the Commission on
Accreditation, meeting in Philadelphia, Pennsylvania, adopted
educational standards, a statement on policies and procedures

and several other guidelines and statements. The process for the validation of the standards commenced.

The Straight Chiropractic Academic Standards Association was formed in order to adopt and promulgate academic standards for straight chiropractic education. The chiropractic profession has no claim to any other accreditation qualification.[3]''

Accreditation, with its support of the taxpayer in education, may at long last end the controversy.

On one hand is the Straight Chiropractic Academic Standards Association Committee on Accreditation as an accrediting body espousing the sole objective of removing interferences to the body's own propensity to heal itself. Which interprets to mean the practice of spinal adjustments to release interference on the nervous system allowing the natural innate forces within the body to heal itself.

On the other hand is the Council on Chiropractic Education with the objective of educating the chiropractic physician, and in my opinion, invading the practice field of medicine and physical therapy without meeting the established accrediting standards of these professions.

Championed by the Federation of Straight Chiropractic Organizations (FSCO), Thom Gelardi, D.C., President of Sherman College of Straight Chiropractic, Pennsylvania College of Straight Chiropracitc and others of us who were not only dedicated but determined that chiropractic education must be confined within its own separate and distinct principles and practice, a continuing action program was undertaken to secure the new accrediting agency.

Opposed on every hand by the colleges and organizations which supported and had fled to the Council on Chiropractic Education (CCE) when that organization was recognized by the United States Department of Education in 1974, the task appeared insuperable.

But August, 1988, witnessed the victory when the announcement was made to the membership by the Federation of Straight Chiropractic Organizations:

> *"It gives me great pleasure to announce the approval of the Straight Chiropractic Academic Standards Association (SCASA) by the United States Department of Education."*

Chiropractic within the confines of its own principles and practice could now enter the mainstream of education based on a legally sound, separate and distinct school in the healing arts.

> *"We have seen the Future and it is now,"* wrote Joseph F. Donofrio, D.C., *Chairman of the Federation of Straight Chiropractic Organizations (FSCO), as he made the announcement to the membership.*

The approval of the Straight Chiropractic Academic Standards Association (SCASA) by the United States Department of Education stands with little question as one of the most significant, far-reaching gains to the professional advancement of chiropractic.

For educational recognition allows chiropractic to move forward in service to humanity within its own field of practice.

As a contrast under the heading 'Curriculum' in the Education Standards for Chiropractic Colleges, March, 1978, The Council on Chiropractic Education is this wording:

Curriculum

''The purpose of the curriculum is to provide the means for giving a student a thorough understanding of the structure and function of the human organism in health and disease. A well-balanced presentation should give the student an understanding of the essential features of the life processes; digestion, excretion, physical and mental growth, nutrition, metabolism, energy, nervous control, the significance of developmental defects, behavior, and other elements which are fundamental of the understanding of pathological conditions. An understanding of structure and functions should make it possible for students to identify deviations from the normal and should provide the essential facts required later for the diagnosis, prognosis, and treatment of disease.[4]''

Chiropractic is a separate, not duplicated nor duplicating practice in the healing arts. And accreditation assures the general public, the educational community, governmental and private agencies that an institution meets established quality standards.

The Commission on Accreditation of the Straight Chiropractic Academic Standards Association is a legitimate accrediting agency for the chiropractic profession. These standards assure quality training for chiropractors keeping within the profession's own principles and practice.

The use of our tax dollars to teach medical and physical therapy practices to students enrolled in chiropractic colleges is not only the ultimate insult to the role of chiropractic as founded and envisioned by the Palmers, but it also raises the question: ''Is this a right use of our tax dollars in furthering education?''

I have every confidence, as the facts are known, taxpayers and the public will demand that no monies be allocated in any manner to educate the chiropractor to practice medical, physical therapy, or any other practice foreign to chiropractic.

One must also ask: "Will the chiropractic profession take the necessary action to correct this intolerable situation or must others do it for us?" The attempt to accomplish "dual accreditation" without meeting the long-existing standards of the medical and physical therapy professions hangs like the Sword of Damocles over each and every member of the profession.

The Straight Chiropractic Academic Standards Association Commission on Accreditation offers the hope that chiropractic will be recognized and accredited within its legitimate confines and in so doing will be able to take its place in the educational community as a separate, distinct profession.

"The stanglehold that the 'mixer' oriented Council on Chiropractic Education (CCE), has held on chiropractic education for the past fourteen years has been broken with the recognition of the Straight Chiropractic Academic Standards Association, (SCASA). The action is one of the most significant happenings in chiropractic," said George B. Banks, D.C.*

"As a past President of the Palmer College of Chiropractic Alumni Association, I am acutely aware of many of the problems facing the profession, the new graduate, and, as well as those who may be considering chiropractic as a career. With this accrediting approval, I firmly believe that the profession now can look forward to moving into the mainstream of the health professions. In so doing it will gain the respect and confidence it so rightfully deserves."[5]

---

* *George B. Banks, D.C., Salinas, California. Past President of Palmer College Alumni Association, past ICA Board member, Fellow of ICA, Fellow Palmer Academy of Chiropractic.*

References

1. Sherman College of Straight Chiropractic Announcements, 1974, page 5

2. State of Illinois, 84th General Assembly 1985-86

3. Committee on Accreditation of the Straight Chiropractic Academic Standards Association, page 1

4. Educational Standards for Chiropractic Colleges March 1978, The Council on Chiropractic Education

5. Statement of George B. Banks, D.C.

CHAPTER VII

A LOOK AHEAD

What is ahead for chiropractic—what does the future hold? Surely no one is a seer or prophet, but one thing seems a certainty. If the total profession can unite on chiropractic's own principles and practice it can become a major factor in the health science services.

Confucius wrote: "Tis man that makes truth great, not truth that makes man great."

In spite of the conflicts and struggles within the profession, there exists the great truth inherent within the chiropractic principles and practice. And that truth embodied in the principle and practice is that the interference to the flow of impulses over or through the nervous system caused by vertebral subluxations can be released or restored by way of vertebral adjustment. The restoration of an energy impulse flow over or through the nervous system allows for an innate health restoration and maintenance.

The unexplored territory of the spine and the discovery and recognition of an energy impulse flow over or through the nervous system by D. D. Palmer in 1895, has since that time been the subject of endless hours of research by many professions.

It is safe to say that millions of people have benefitted from spinal adjustments. Chiropractic has added millions of years to millions of lives, sparing humanity untold hours of suffering.

Legally, chiropractic is anchored as a separate practice and school in the healing arts. The years ahead should lay further foundations on this fact so that other professions can in no manner make inroads into the field of chiropractic practice without adequate education and licensure.

Actions in malpractice clearly state the separateness of chiropractic as a separate school in the healing arts and allow for chiropractic to be judged by its own standards. Bean, J., in **Wemmett v Mount** (1930), 134 Or 305. 292 P 93, at page 313 said:

> "It is the general rule that in a malpractice action a physician or surgeon is entitled to have his treatment of his patient tested by the rules and principles of the school of medicine to which he belongs, and not by those of some other school, because a person professing to follow one system or school of medicine cannot be expected by his employer to practice any other, and if he performs a treatment with ordinary skill and care in accordance with his system, he is not answerable for bad results. However, the rule, which confines the inquiry as to a practitioner's skill and care to the rules and principles of the school of medicine to which he belongs, does not exclude the testimony of physicians of other schools or experts in other lines when such testimony bears on a point as to which the principles of the schools do or should concur, such as the dangers incident to the use of x-rays, or the existence of a condition that should be recognized by any physician 21 RCL p. 383, 28; **Hilgedorf v Bertschinger** (Or), 285 P 819."

Legislatively, even though some jurisdictions at the present time may hold other practices in a chiropractic legislative act, a concerted action by those dedicated to the separateness of chiropractic from other healing arts, must unite in a total effort to clarify statute language.

Here again legal decisions may well form the basis for action in legislative clarifications. Quoting from a Minnesota Attorney General ruling, 1975:

"Minn Stat 148.01 subd. 1 (1974) defines 'chiropractic' as:...The science of adjusting any abnormal articulations of the human body, especially those of the spinal column, for the purpose of giving freedom of action to impinged nerves that may cause pain or deranged function."

Subdivision 2 declares that the practice of chiropractic is not the practice of medicine, surgery or osteopathy.

*"The (chiropractic) system is well known to the courts, and there are numerous adjudications thereon. **Com. v Zimmerman**, 221 Mass. 184, 108 N.E. 893, Ann Cas. 1916A, 858; **Board of M.E. vs Freenor**, 47 Utah, 430, 154 Pac. 941 Ann. Cas. 1917E, 1156; **Swarts vs Siveny**, 35 R. I. 1, 85 Atl. 33; **State v Johnson**, 84 Kan. 411, 114 Pac. 390, 41 L.R.A. (N.S.) 539: **State vs Gallagher**, 101 Ark.593.143 S. W. 98, 38 L.R.A. (N.S.) 328 and other cases cited in L.R.A. 1917 C, 823."* The Massachusetts Supreme Court in **Zimmerman** described the technique of chiropractic adjustments as follows:

"In making 'adjustments', the patient was placed on a low table with face downward and the vertebra which was out of condition was given a quick thrust or push by the hands of the defendant. The acts performed by the defendant constitute, first an examination of the vertebrae of the spinal column and a determination whether they are in a normal or in an unnatural position; and, second, a manipulation of such of the vertebrae as are found to be out of position, so that they will become regular and correct with reference to each other. 108 N. E. at 894."

The foregoing indicates that the common meaning and understanding of 'adjustment' at the time that term was defined by the legislature in 1919 was limited to manipulations of joints, especially those of the spinal column.

When construing the limited scope of practice of health care professionals, courts have uniformly applied the principle that the words of a statute must be interpreted in the sense in which they were understood at the time the law was enacted. After citing several sources discussing interpretations of 'chiropractic' similar to that given in the **Zimmerman** case, **supra**, the court in **People vs Fowler**, 32 Cal. App. 2d Supp. 737, 84 P2d 326 (1938), stated:

"This general consensus of definitions, current at and before the time the Chiropractic Act was adopted, shows what was meant by the term 'chiropractic' when used in that act. 'The words of a statute must be taken in the sense in which they were understood at the time when the statute was enacted.' 25 R.C.L. 959; **Werner vs Hillman, etc., Co.**, 1930, 300 Pa. 256, 150 A. 471, 70 A.L.R. 967, 970; **Dunn vs Commissioner**, 1933, 281 Mass. 376, 183 N.E. 889, 87 A.L.R. 998, 1002, 84 P2d 331. See also **Cress v California State Board of Medical Examiners**, 213 Cal. app. 2d 195, 28 Cal. Rptr. 621 (1963); **United States vs 22 Devices, More or Less, Halox Therapeutic Generator**, 98 F. Supp. 914 (S.D. Cal. 1951). **State ex rel Wheat vs Moore**, 154 Kan. 193, 117 P2d 598 (1941); **Ingebritson vs Tjernlund Manufacturing Company**, 289 Minn. 232, 183 N. W. 2d 552 (1971)."

As the facts are known, education too, will have a major impact on the future of the profession. I believe the state and federal government will ultimately withdraw funds from any chiropractic college teaching the practice of other professions and failing to meet legitimate accrediting standards for those professional practices. Chiropractic colleges will then confine their teaching and practice to chiropractic principles and practice. The years ahead will, in my opinion, witness the demise of the mixer chiropractic colleges and the mixer chiropractic physician. The long-held "mixer" and "straight" connotations will be of the past. Chiropractors will be chiropractors.

Research will dominate chiropractic activity as the principles and practice are further validated. This basic physiological function of the role of the nervous system gives rise to a most worthwhile research program for the profession.

A nerve could be compared to a telephone cable. Thousands of axons are inside the nerve cable. These axons could be compared to individual telephone wires. Each axon is "hooked up" to the brain which is the innate, intelligent, power source. Each axon is capable of carrying a message or impulse destined for a muscle or other tissue cells. This impulse, measurable, but in the late Dr. B. J. Palmer Chiropractic Research Clinic never found to be over 5/1 millionth of a volt, is sent efferently over the axon or nerve fiber causing a contraction of the muscle fiber or other action in the tissue cells.

A corresponding energy impulse flow is returned to the brain by the afferent energy flow cycle. The innate intelligence within the brain is thus kept informed as to the needs, demands and condition of body function.

The energy impulse message flow over the nervous system must not be interrupted if normal, coordinated function is to take place in the body. For this is how the innate intelligence located in the brain of each living organism communicates with the body. Maintaining this 'cycle of life' free from interference will be the continuing challenge of research.

Today too, this question is raised in many minds. How do drugs affect the nervous system? This question was studied in 1961, by Dr. B. J. Palmer in the B. J. Palmer Chiropractic Research Clinic:

> *"The electroencephaloneuromentimpograph pickup will average generally five-one millionth of a volt. That is assuming that the impulse supply is flowing normally and freely. Under stimulation such as whiskey, rye, beer, other liquors, and other methods of electrical treatments or stimulation, it will climb above the graph scale. Under depressant drugs such as morphine, cocaine, novacaine, or other drugs of like purpose, graph readings show a below normal impulse graph value flow.*[3]*"*

Research such as this can be of immeasurable help in finding a solution to the ongoing drug abuse problem in our society.

Preventative health care and services are no doubt to be one of the major roles of the healing professions in the years ahead. The services will be those not only to get well but to stay well. Preventative health care is paramount in the services to be provided. Chiropractic can play a major role in these services by keeping the nervous system free of interruption and interferences. This is basic to a normal functioning of the body. All tax supported institutions dedicated to helping sick people get well should utilize the services chiropractic has to offer. And all professionals should cooperate in the best interest of patient health.

There is little question but that chiropractic will continue to have a major impact in the understanding of the role and functioning of the nervous system.

The words of Liddon express my feelings of the profession regarding research.

"The restless mind of man cannot but press a principle to the real limits of its applicaton, even though centuries should intervene between the premises and the conclusion.⁴"

Researchers in vertebral adjusting, those such as— Ralph Gregory, D.C. and James W. Young, D.C. will continue to lead the way toward more exact specific spinal adjustive technics to release interferences from the nervous system due to spinal subluxations.

The years ahead may well see science and the scientific researcher turn away from drugs, chemicals and experimental surgery and look within each individual to find the causative factors for dis-ease and sickness.

Could it be that this 'discovery' by D. D. Palmer be utilized to its fullest and be this new direction for research in helping humanity enjoy a fuller, richer life? Chiropractic offers this hope.

Generations are as the days of toilsome mankind. What a father has made, the son can make and enjoy, but he has also work of his own appointed to him. Thus all things wax and roll onwards—arts, establishments, opinions, nothing is ever completed, but completing.⁵

Those of us who laid the foundation for chiropractic in legal recognition, in legislative recognition, the inclusion of chiropractic in insurance, and industry, health and welfare plans as well as many, many other areas within its true scope of practice are grateful for the opportunity that was ours. It is our hope that the groundwork in which we so actively participated will hasten the day when chiropractic services are available to all people.

But a warning and admonition was given the profession by the late Dr. John Q. Thaxton, the second president of the International Chiropractic Association when he said:

"Unless the chiropractic profession confines its practice within its own principles and practice, it does not deserve to be a separate profession." Our experience echoes this thought.

And someday, too, humanity may know the depth of understanding propounded by D. D. Palmer when he stated of his discovery:

"It is destined to revolutionize the theory and practice of the healing arts.[6]*"*

John D. Rockefeller, Sr., after he had established the Foundation for Medical Research bearing his name, must have communed with Nature for, when nearing the century mark in age, he designated her as the Great Physician.

"Men who are studying the problem of disease tell us that it is becoming more and more evident that the forces which conquer sickness are within the body itself, and that it is only when they are reduced below the normal that disease can get a foothold. The way to ward off disease therefore," he continues, *"is to tone up the body generally, and when disease has secured a foothold, the way to combat it is to help those natural resisting agencies that are within the body itself.*[7]*"*

In his book Bacteria Inc., Cash Asher also writes:

"The over-emphasis on artificial procedures, combined with the false belief that scientific medicine has made it safe to disregard the laws of Nature, hangs over the human race like the Sword of Damocles.[8]"

Millions of people travel the road of life never realizing the importance of the spine in sickness and health. In the years ahead as chiropractors all over the world concentrate their efforts totally on the location and adjustment of vertebral subluxations, chiropractic services in health care will become as common and acceptable as medical practice or any of the other valued health services. Chiropractors will adopt a scope of practice in keeping with chiropractic principles. As the role of chiropractic becomes the chiropractic role, the spine, the literal switchboard of the nervous system, will become a signal area of first importance in health restoration and maintenance as vertebrae are kept in their normal position through spinal adjustments. This because spinal subluxations disturb the normal function of the central nervous system and in so doing disrupt normal body function.

Many years ago I attended a term at Willamette University in Salem, Oregon before beginning my chiropractic career. Dr. Bruce Baxter was then the President of the University. I will always remember a quotation which he recited during the chapel assembly. He said:

"A sane philosophy of life is a precious possession and that escape from the despotism of authority into the privilege of thinking for one's self is a priceless accomplishment."

This philosophy of chiropractic—the knowledge—is

too, a priceless possession. The essence of that knowledge is that the innate energy flow of energy over the nervous system from brain to body and body to brain must not be disrupted, interfered with, or disturbed if health is to be restored and maintained.

This is the principle, the Law of Life as given the world by the three generations of Palmers, D. D., B. J. and David, as each in his own allotted time carried the message inherent within that fragile truth.

The application and the means to accomplish its purpose will be pursued by generations and for generations.

In the end, as the knowledge inherent within that truth becomes common knowledge to all, mankind will live a more normal, healthier life—freed of the artificialities in trying to regain and maintain health. Health is the birthright of each individual—and health and healing come from within.

Chiropractic will never be 'sold' on words or on advertising to a waiting people. Chiropractic will only be 'sold' on deeds, on its merits—on proof that vertebral adjusting proves its true worth in releasing the imprisoned impulses caused by the vertebral subluxation this in turn allowing for a normal sustained energy flow over the nervous system for innate health restoration and maintenance.

For chiropractors will never fool the public into thinking they are Doctors of Medicine, Osteopathy, Physical Therapists or other professionals.

Too long the public has had access to first-rate services from those professions to be fooled by a chiropractic licentiate attempting to emulate the medical doctor, the physiotherapist or other professions.

Chiropractic blazes a new trail bringing attention to

the spine and nervous system and what can happen when vertebral subluxations are adjusted.

On the other hand, it is my firm conviction that chiropractors will guard zealously the gains that were made in establishing chiropractic as a separate school and practice in the healing arts.

If medical, physical therapy, osteopathic or other practitioners attempt to practice chiropractic without qualifications, it is my opinion that chiropractors will rise to the occasion and not permit such to happen.

But further, the future may well see chiropractic statute language in all jurisdictions defined within its own scope of practice and practitioners of other healing arts prohibited from practicing chiropractic without qualifications.

Time moves on. The question moves—as does the answer. And this is the question.

"Can the chiropractic profession confine itself within its own principles and practice until all humanity may have access to the vertebral subluxation—vertebral adjustment principle of health restoration? This can become a reality only when the role of chiropractic becomes the chiropractor's role.

That epochal event on September 18, 1895, which restored hearing to a man who had waited in silence for seventeen years has given humanity this truism.

Generated within the brain is an energy which flows over the nerve pathways. Extending from tiny cells in the brain is a nerve fiber connecting each with a corresponding tissue cell of the body and from the tissue cell is also a nerve pathway back to its controlling brain cell. Over this nerve pathway flows the energy or mental impulse which is the 'spark of life'—with it, the tissue cell functions. Without it—normal function is absent. Over and above all of this is an inborn intelligence which coordinates, directs and controls these billions of cells in their activity for coordinated function or health. The Pathway to Health is a nervous system free of pressure allowing a normal energy flow from the brain to the body at all times.

A vertebral subluxation in the spinal column occludes a foramen, that occlusion produces pressure on nerves. That pressure on nerves interferes with the normal quantity transmission of mental impulse flow between brain and body, and in exact ratio as that mental impulse flow is decreased at the periphery, dis-ease is created and increased in the same ratio.

By spinal adjustment, the vertebral subluxation is restored to normal position. This takes pressure off the nervous system allowing for a normal mental impulse flow over the nervous system. In exact ratio as that mental impulse flow is restored at the periphery, dis-ease is decreased and health restored.

References

1. Supreme Court of the State of Oregon. March Term 1956. Jessie Fern Sheppard vs P. B. Firth, D. C. p. 38.

2. State of Minnesota, Office Attorney General Mar. 10, 1975 p. 6-7-8

3. The B. J. Palmer Chiropractic Research Clinic, Davenport, Iowa, XXXIX

4. The New Dictionary of Thoughts, originally compiled by Tyron Edwards, A. M.
   Enlarged by C. N. Catrevas, A. B. Jonathan Edwards, A. M. Ralph Emerson Browns, A.M. p. 520

5. The New Dictionary of Thoughts, originally compiled by Tyron Edwards, A.M. (Carlyle)
   Enlarged by C. N. Catrevas, A. B. Jonathan Edwards, A. M. Ralph Emerson Browns, A. M. p. 524

6. The Science, Art and Philsophy of Chiropractic by D. D. Palmer

7. Bacteria Inc., Cash Asher, 1949 p. 103-4

8. Bacteria Inc., Cash Asher, 1949 p. 108

_____APPENDIX_____

A. **Neuroanatomy of Hearing**
A 1. **Nelson v. Harrington**
B. **Legal Decisions and Comments**

(A)

NEUROANATOMY OF HEARING

The acoustic or auditory or eighth cranial nerve is made up of afferent fibers from the internal ear which are arranged in two sets: (1) the vestibular part (or vestibular nerve) is concerned with equilibration and from its nuclei in the pons some fibers extend to the cerebellum and others pass down the spinal cord to form connections with motor centers of the spinal nerves; and (2) the cochlear part (or cochlear nerve) is concerned with hearing. The fibers of the cochlear nerve are bipolar and arise from the spiral ganglion situated in the inner ear. These cells send one fiber toward the brain in the acoustic nerve and the other to end in terminal arborizations around the hair cells of the organ of Corti.

The acoustic center in the brain is located in the temporal lobe of the cerebrum. Destruction of both acoustic centers will result in total deafness, whereas, if only one center is destroyed, the result is impaired hearing. This may be explained by the fact that some of the nerve fibers arising from one ear may cross over within the neuron pathways and become a part of the opposite cochlear nerve—an arrangement similar to that found in the optic chiasma of the visual apparatus.

The cochlear nerve has both reflex connections in the brain stem, and cortical connections through the lateral lemniscus, medial geniculate body of the thalamus and auditory radiations for conscious sensations of hearing.

It is often pointed out by those who would deny the science of chiropractic that the acoustic nerve does not leave the cranial vault and thus it could not be subject to nerve interference from a vertebral subluxation. It is anatomically true that the acoustic nerve is located wholly within the cranium. However, there are connections to this nerve from nerves which are situated in areas subject to nerve interference from vertebral subluxations as we know them.

Of particular interest is the superior cervical ganglion located behind the carotid sheath, and opposite the transverse processes of atlas, axis and 3rd cervical vertebra.

This is the uppermost ganglion of a series which are joined to each other by intervening nerve cords and collectively these make up the gangliated trunk of the sympathetic nervous system.

This system lies partly in front of and to either side of the vertebral column and extends from the ganglion impar in front of the coccyx to the ganglion surrounding the anterior communicating artery of the brain (Ribes ganglion).

The superior cervical ganglion gives off nerve branches which help form the carotid plexus; and other branches from the plexus are considered to control the blood supply to the ear.

One particularly large branch is known as the internal carotid nerve which accompanies the internal carotid artery. As the artery ascends through the base of the skull, the nerve breaks up into several branches that form the internal carotid plexus. This plexus gives branches to the tympanic nerve.

Certain mental impulses originating in the brain and passing downward through the spinal cord are able to communicate with the gangliated chain of the sympathetic system by way of the rami communicates. The rami are short, thread-like connections between the anterior divisions of the spinal nerves and the sympathetic chain ganglia. They may be regarded as visceral branches of the nerves. There are two types (a) white communicating rami, which pass from the spinal cord to the sympathetic chain ganglia, and, (b) gray communicating rami, that pass from cells in the sympathetic-chain ganglia to the anterior divisions of the spinal nerves. The cervical nerves have only gray rami connected with them, and the thoracic and upper lumbar nerves have both white and gray rami.

A vertebral subluxation may interfere with the flow of mental impulses to and through the gangliated chain by exerting interference either in the spinal cord, the spinal nerve or the ganglion itself. It is entirely possible that these are trophic impulses which supply the structures of the internal ear, and that interference with their flow will result in nutritional disturbances to the parts supplied by them.

Neurological evidence indicates that in addition to the branches of the carotid plexus the ear is also supplied by the tympanic branch of the glossopharyngeal nerve (Jacobson's nerve), and the auriculotemporal branch of the trigeminal. Each of these nerves has a similar connection with pathways via the gangliated chain of the sympathetic system.

(A1)

NELSON v. HARRINGTON
72 Wisc 591, 40 N. W. 228 (1888)

1. Malpractice—Clairvoyants—Degree Of Care And Skill.

In an action against a clairvoyant physician for malpractice, the court was asked to charge that if, at the time defendant was called to treat plaintiff, both parties understood that he would treat him according to the approved practice of clairvoyant physicians, and that he did so treat him, with the ordinary skill and knowledge of the clairvoyant system, plaintiff could not recover. Held properly refused. Instead of the words, "with the ordinary skill and knowledge of the clairvoyant system," the instructions should have read, "with the ordinary skill and knowledge of physicians in good standing, practicing in that vicinity." One who holds himself out as a healer of diseases must, no matter to what particular school or system he belongs, be held to the duty of reasonable skill, in the light of the present state of medical science.

2. Same—Imputed Negligence—Parent And Child.

Defendant cannot be heard to charge that the father of plaintiff, a minor, was negligent, in that he employed defendant to treat his son with full knowledge of defendant's methods of diagnosis and prescription.

3. Evidence—Depositions In Another Case.

Defendant offered in evidence a deposition of plaintiff's father taken in a case brought by the latter against defendant for loss of his son's services caused by the malpractice complained of in this action. Held properly excluded; it being the statement of a witness made at a different time and place, in a different cause, and clearly inadmissible as evidence in chief against plaintiff.

4. Trial—Misconduct Of Counsel.

Plaintiff's counsel having commenced to comment to the jury on the fact that defendant and certain physicians present had not been called by defendant as witnesses, the court expressed its disapprobation of this line of remark, and in the general charge instructed the jury not to draw any presumption from the fact that those persons were not called. Held, that defendant was not prejudiced.

5. Same

On the trial it was shown that defendant placed "Dr." on his sign and prescriptions. Counsel for defendant remarked in argument that when he did that he violated the laws of Wisconsin. Held, that the remark was not serious, even if not true.

Appeal from circuit court, Dane County.

This is an action brought by Thomas Nelson, by guardian ad litem, against Charles F. Harrington, to recover damages for the alleged malpractice of the defendant as a physician. The substance of the complaint is that for several years before September, 1885, the defendant had been engaged in the practice of medicine and surgery in the city of Madison, and during all that time, advertised and held himself out to the public as a physician, and attended to all such diseases and ailments of the human body as a physician is usually called upon to treat, and such as are ordinarily treated by physicians

of good standing and repute in said city of Madison; that
he also gave out that he possessed some mysterious
power, insight, or skill, not possessed by physicians in
general, and for that reason could cure diseases generally thought to be incurable, and could relieve ordinary
diseases and ailments more speedily and effectually than
other physicians in good standing and repute as such;
that shortly before September 1, 1885, the plaintiff,
Thomas Nelson, (then about 15 years of age) was
afflicted with some disease of his right hip, and on or
about that date his father called the defendant, as such
physician, to attend him, and treat him for said disease;
that the defendant undertook to attend the plaintiff as a
physician, and treat and care for him in a proper manner
as such physician, but that, disregarding his duty in the
premises, the defendant wrongfully and carelessly failed
to make a proper or ordinary examination of the plaintiff,
such as a physician of ordinary skill, care, or prudence
would have made, and pronounced said disease to be
rheumatism when it was in fact a disease of the hip joint,
which disease has well-known, peculiar signs and symptoms, which a physician of ordinary skill and care would
at once detect; that there are well-known and acknowl-
edged remedies for such disease, which all physicians of
ordinary skill and prudence invariably use in the treatment thereof; that the defendant, in disregard of his duty
as such physician, negligently and unskillfully treated the
plaintiff for rheumatism, and not hip-joint disease, and
continued so to treat him until about the middle of the
following January; that during such time the defendant
encouraged the plaintiff to walk persistently, and use his
right leg in walking, asserting that walking was beneficial

to him; that the plaintiff grew constantly worse under such treatment, until he could not walk, and suffered great pain and distress during the time, but the defendant constantly asserted, when told he was getting worse, that he was in fact getting better; that in January, 1886, after the plaintiff had wholly lost the use of his leg, other physicians were called in, and by most persistent and thorough medical treatment the plaintiff, to some extent, recovered the use of his leg, but will be a cripple for life; that, if the defendant had treated the plaintiff properly, he would have been speedily and completely restored to health, and would have recovered the full use of his leg; also that he would have been relieved in a great measure from the suffering he was compelled to endure. The defendant answered that, during the time stated in the complaint, he had been what is commonly known and understood as a spiritualist and clairvoyant physician, and, as such, has treated diseases and ailments of the human body, and prescribed for patients calling upon him for treatment; most of his practice having been in and about the city of Madison. The anwser proceeds as follows: "That on the 1st day of September, 1885, the said plaintiff, in person or by his father, Tollef A. Nelson, called upon this defendant for treatment for some ailment of which he, the said plaintiff, was then suffering; but defendant alleges that whatever treatment he gave the said plaintiff was strictly in accordance with the ordinary and customary practice and system of practice as used and employed by spiritualists and clairvoyants in diagnosing, attending, and prescribing for diseases and ailments of the human body, and that he was employed by the said plaintiff and the said Tollef A. Nelson to treat

the said Thomas Nelson only as a spiritualist and clairvoyant, and not in any manner as an ordinary physician
or surgeon possessed of the ordinary knowledge or skill
belonging to physicians and surgeons and doctors of
medicine in the regular schools of practice; that the said
Tollef A. Nelson and the said Thomas Nelson both well
knew the manner of diagnosing and prescribing for diseases employed by this defendant, and well knew that
this defendant employed no other and had no other
manner or method of determining or diagnosing diseases and ailments of the human body before the said
plaintiff came to this defendant; that said plaintiff came
to this defendant desiring and expecting this defendant
to diagnose said disease, and prescribe for the same as a
spiritualist and clairvoyant physician. Defendant further
alleges, on information and belief, that the said Thomas
Nelson was, at the time of said treatment, afflicted with
some rheumatic affection of his limb and hip, from which
he had been suffering for a long time prior to calling this
defendant to treat said ailment." The cause was tried by
a jury, and resulted in a verdict and judgment for the
plaintiff. The testimony and proceedings upon the trial,
so far as the same are essential to an understanding of
the exceptions considered, are sufficiently stated in the
opinion. The defendant appeals from the judgment.

Rogers & Hall, for appellant. *Pinney & Sanborn,* for
respondent.

Lyon, J., *(after stating the facts as above.)* The question has
been raised whether this is an action for the breach of a
contract, or one sounding in tort, for the alleged unskillful
and negligent manner in which the defendant, as a physi-

cian, performed his duty to the plaintiff. Although the complaint alleges the implied contract of the defendant to treat the plaintiff in a skillful and proper manner, yet the *gravamen* of the action is alleged to be that the defendant disregarded his duty in the premises by negligently, wrongfully, and carelessly failing to make a proper diagnosis of the plaintiff's disease, and to prescribe proper remedies therefor. These allegations characterize the action. They show it to be solely for a breach of defendant's duty as a physician, founded upon his legal obligations as such, without reference to the implied contract. The contract is stated in the complaint as mere matter of inducement, and might as well have been omitted. It must be held, therefore, that the action is for the breach of duty—the negligence and wrong—and not upon contract. *Wood vs Railway Co.*, 32 Wis. 398. The general rule of law is that a physician or surgeon, or one who holds himself out as such, whether duly licensed or not, when he accepts an employment to treat a patient professionally, must exercise such reasonable care and skill in that behalf as is usually possessed and exercised by physicians or surgeons in good standing, of the same system or school of practice, in the vicinity or locality of his practice, having due regard to the advanced state of medical or surgical science at the time. This rule is elementary. It has its foundation in most persuasive considerations of public policy. Its purpose is to protect the health and lives of the public, particularly of the weak or credulous, the ignorant or unwise, from the unskillfulness of negligence of medical practitioners, by holding such practitioners liable to respond in damages for the results of their unskillfulness or negligence. Citation of authority to support the rule would be superfluous. It was substantially (perhaps not so fully) laid down and applied in *Gates vs Fleischer*, 67 Wis. 504, 30 N.W. Rep. 674, and is sustained by numerous cases, many of which are cited in the briefs of counsel on both sides.

The defendant is what is known as a "clairvoyant physician," and held himself out, as other physicians do, as competent to treat disease of the human system. He did not belong to, or practice in accordance with the rules of, any existing school of physicians, governed by formulated rules for treating diseases and injuries, to which rules all practitioners of that school are supposed to adhere. The testimony shows that his mode of diagnosis and treatment consisted in voluntarily going into a sort of trance condition, and while in such condition to give a diagnosis of the case, and prescribe for the ailment of the patient thus disclosed. He made no personal examination, applied no tests to discover the malady, and resorted to no other source of information as to the past or present condition of the plaintiff. Indeed, he did not profess to have been educated in the science of medicine. He trusted implicitly to the accuracy of his diagnosis thus made, and of his prescriptions thus given.

The general rule above stated requires of one holding himself out as a physician the exercise of the same skill and care as is ordinarily exercised by physicians in good standing, who belong to the same school of medicine, and practice under the same rule. To constitute a school of medicine under this rule, it must have rules and principles of practice for the guidance of all its members, as respects principles, diagnosis, and remedies, which each member is supposed to observe in any given case. Thus, any competent practitioner of any given school would treat a given case substantially the same as any other competent practitioner of the same school would treat it. One school may believe in the potency of drugs and blood-letting, and another may believe in the principle *similia similibus curantur*; still others may believe in the potency of water, or of roots and herbs; yet each school has its own peculiar principles and rules for the government of its practitioners in the treatment of diseases. Not so, however, with the clairvoyant practice. True, the practice has but one mode of ascertaining what the disease is, and the remedy therefore. This mode has already been stated. But the mode in which a physician acquires a knowledge of his profession has nothing to do with his school or system of practice. One person may acquire such knowledge from certain books; another from certain other books, which perhaps teach different principles; still another from oral communication, as lectures, et cet., or from experience alone; and still another from his intuition when in an abnormal mental state; yet these differences do not necessarily constitute separate schools of medicine. The clairvoyant and the practitioner of the allopathic or homeopathic system may belong to the same school or system, provided they adopt the same principles and observe the same rules of treatment. The methods by which a man acquires a knowledge of medical science is one thing, and the principles and rules which govern him in the practice of medicine is another and very different thing. This is just the difference between clairvoyant physicians as a class and the practitioners of a school or system of medical practice recognized in the general rule of professional ability above laid down. The regular physician of any school or system acquires his professional knowledge by the study of the general principles of the science, and applies such knowledge to each particular case as it arises, while the clairvoyant physician may have no such general knowledge, but believes himself especially and effectually educated to treat each particular case as it is presented to him, without reference to any particular system or school. These observations dispose of the exceptions based upon the rejection of testimony offered to show that the defendant practiced only as a clairvoyant physician. That was conclusively proved before, and the rejection of the testimony (if material under other circumstances) was of no importance. It should be observed that the answer of the defendant does not allege, and no testimony was given or offered to show, that clairvoyant physicians, as a class, treat diseases upon any such principles, or that rules have been formulated which each practitioner is supposed to follow in the treatment of disease, as in the case with the schools or systems of medicine before mentioned. Clairvoyant physicians have a common mode of acquiring their knowledge of cases, but their methods of treatment may be contradictory, and as numerous as are the practitioners, and no principle or rule of clairvoyant treatment be violated thereby. The proposition that one holding himself out as a medical practitioner, and as competent to treat human maladies, who accepts a person as a patient, and treats him for disease, may, because he resorts to some peculiar method of determining the nature of the disease and the remedy therefore, be exonerated from all liability for unskillfulness on his part, no matter how serious the consequences may be, cannot be entertained. The proposition, if accepted as true, would, as already suggested, contravene a sound public policy. It matters not that the patient, or those who are responsible for him, know the methods of the practitioner. The responsibility for malpractice must still be laid on the latter. It should be stated in this connection that the father of the plaintiff, who employed the defendant to treat his son, testified that he so employed him because he believed him to be a skillful physician; that he did not depend upon the trance business, but on the defendant, the same as he would on any other physician; and that he believed in him because he had performed remarkable cures. It follows that the court properly refused to give an instruction proposed on behalf of the defendant in these words: "If defendant was a clairvoyant physician, and professed and held himself out to be such, and the plaintiff and his parents knew it, and at the time he was called to treat the plaintiff both parties understood and expected that he would treat him according to the approved practice of clairvoyant physicians, and that he did so treat him, and in strict accordance with the clairvoyant system of practice, and with the ordinary skill and knowledge of that system, then the plaintiff cannot recover, and your verdict must be for the defendant." Instead of the words, "with the ordinary skill and knowledge of that system," employed therein, it should have read, "with the ordinary skill and knowledge of physicians in good standing, practicing in that vicinity."

Since the cause was argued our attention has been called to the late case of *Wheeler vs Sawyer*, decided by the supreme judicial court of Maine, and reported in 15 Atl. Rep. 67. The statutes of Maine allow any person to prac-

tice medicine who has obtained from the municipal officers of the town in which he resides a certificate of good
moral character. The plaintiff had such certificate, and
practiced according to the principles and methods of
those calling themselves "Christian Scientists." The case
shows that practitioners of "Christian Science" use no
medicine, and the plaintiff used none. It has now become
common knowledge that their treatment is entirely mental. The action was for professional services. The objections to a recovery were "that the so-called 'Christian
Science' is a delusion; that its principles and methods are
absurd; that its professors are charlatans; that no patient
can possibly be benefitted by their treatment." The court
held all this immaterial, and said, in substance, that the
patient got all he bargained for, and must pay for it at the
agreed price. There is no question of liability for malpractice in the case. On the contrary, the patient said he was
improved under the treatment. Were the defendant in
the present case authorized by law to practice medicine,
and should a patient employ him to go into a clairvoyant
state, and while in such state to tell him his malady and
the remedy therefore, and agree to pay him a certain
sum of money for such services, and were the defendant
to render the service, doing the patient no injury, but a
benefit rather, an action brought by the defendant to
recover the stipulated compensation would be like the
Maine case. We perceive no valid objection to a recovery
by the plaintiff in either case. It goes without saying that
we have here no such case for determination, and the
Maine adjudication does not aid us. We have not been
referred to any case in the books of an action for malpractice against a clairvoyant physician, (so-called,) and

have found none. It is cause for surprise if no such case has arisen; for it is believed that this method has been employed quite extensively for many years, in different parts of the country. Whether the absence of such cases is to be accounted for on the theory that the bar and public have generally believed that this class of physicians are not legally responsible for want of skill, or because no member of it has been guilty of malpractice, or upon some other theory, is not here determined. Probably the fact that such cases have not come before the courts is not very significant. For want of them, however, we have been compelled to decide this case solely in the light of elementary rules of law, which perhaps furnish just as safe a basis for judgment. In this connection brief reference will be made to a case cited by counsel for defendant in his argument which then impressed us as being nearer in point than any other case cited. It is that of *McKleroy vs Sewell*, 73 Ga. 657. The court sustained an instruction to the jury in these words: "If a man sends for a doctor, and the doctor treats the patient while he, the doctor, is intoxicated, and the patient afterwards calls in said doctor, and continues to employ him, it would be a waiver of all objections to the doctor on account of his habit of intoxication." The language of this instruction (copied in the brief of counsel) seemed broad enough to cut off an action for malpractice. On looking into the case, however, we find that action, like the Maine case, was by a physician to recover for professional services. The court said: "Surely, one cannot object to a doctor's bill on account of past intoxication, when he treats him as a family physician for years afterwards." It is strongly intimated in that case that the defendant might recoup in the action for damages caused by malpractice. If so, he might maintain an independent action for such damages. Hence the case is not in point, and throws no light on the present case.

The claim that the defendant belonged to and treated the plaintiff in accordance with the principles and rules of a particular school of medicine, and is relieved from liability in this action because thereof, having been negatived, the law applicable to the case may, we think, be correctly summarized as follows: One who holds himself out as a healer of diseases, and accepts employment as such, must be held to the duty of reasonable skill in the exercise of his vocation. Failing in this, he must be held liable for any damages proximately caused by unskillful treatment of his patient. This is simply applying the rule of liability to which all persons are subject who hold themselves out, and accept employment, as experts In any profession, art, or trade. The theory upon which an expert practices his profession, art, or trade, the sources from whence he derives his knowledge of it, the tools and appliances he employs in the exercise of his calling, his methods of work, are not controlling considerations. The courts pass no judgment upon these matters. They look only to results. Thus, a person may rely entirely upon his genius, or normal intuitions, for some line of mechanical work, and hold himself out as an expert, and accept employment therein, without previous training or practice. The law holds him responsible if he does his work unskillfully, although he does the best he can. He takes the risks of the quality or accuracy of his genius or intuitions. On the same principle one who holds himself out as a medical expert, and accepts employment as a healer of diseases, but who relies exclusively for diagnosis and remedies upon some occult influence exerted upon him, or some mental intuition received by him, when in an abnormal condition, in like manner takes the risks of the quality or accuracy of such influence or intuition. If these move him so imperfectly or inaccurately that, although he pursues the course of treatment thus pointed out or indicated to him, if he fails to treat the patient with reasonable skill, he is liable for the consequences. The only difference in the two cases is, the mechanic acts under normal, and the physician under abnormal, influence or intuition. The law does not concern itself with the quality of the mechanic's genius, or with the reality or nature of such alleged occult influence or intuition which controls the physician in his treatment of his patient. It only takes cognizance of the question, did the practitioner or expert render the service he undertook in a reasonably skillful manner? That question, as applied to the defendant, the jury, upon sufficient proof, have answered in the negative.

As to the alleged negligence of the defendant in his treatment of the plaintiff, it is enough to say that any person who is legally responsible for his conduct is liable for all damages suffered by another which are the proximate result of his negligence or want of ordinary care. Of course, the defendant is subject to this rule; and here it may be observed that negligence cannot properly be imputed to the father of the plaintiff because he employed the defendant to treat his son with full knowledge of the defendant's methods of diagnosis and prescription. At least, the defendant cannot be heard to charge the father with negligence in that behalf. Perhaps a medical practitioner may protect himself from liability for unskillfulness by a special contract that he should not be so liable; but, in the absence of such a contract, the practitioner must be held to his common-law liability. This rule was applied to a common carrier in *Conkey vs Railway Co.*, 31 Wis. 619. Dixon, C. J., there said: "I think, in the absence of special contract or agreement to the contrary, the true policy of the law, now as much as ever, and even more, is to adhere to the strict rules of liability on the part of common carriers established by the common law." Page 633. The reasons which there prevailed for adhering to that rule, and thus vindicating a sound public policy, are much more cogent in the case of the physician, who deals with health and life, instead of property. The charge of the court to the jury, so far as we are able to perceive, is in strict accord with the views herein expressed. It is unnecessary to set it out at length. The testimony tends to show negligence and unskillfulness on the part of the defendant in his treatment of the plaintiff, and supports the verdict. Hence the judgment should not be disturbed unless some material error was committed on the trial. Some of the exceptions have already been determined. Those not passed upon will now be briefly considered. The defendant offered in evidence a deposition of plaintiff's father taken in a case brought by the father against the defendant for loss of his son's services, etc., caused by the same malpractice here complained of. The court rejected the deposition as evidence in chief, but offered to receive it as evidence impeaching the testimony of the father, who had theretofore been examined as a witness on the trial on behalf of the plaintiff. The ruling was clearly right. It was an offer to prove the statements of a witness made at another time and place in a different cause, as evidence in chief against the plaintiff. Of course, such evidence is inadmissible. Certain objections were taken to remarks of counsel in argument. It was proved that the defendant placed the abbreviation "Dr." on his sign and prescriptions. Counsel said that when he did so he violated the laws of Wisconsin. The remark is not a very serious one, at most, even if not true. We think, however, that it is a fair inference from the allegations of the answer, and from the proofs, that the defendant was not a regularly authorized medical practitioner under the laws of this state. The only other objection of this character is that counsel for the plaintiff also commenced to comment to the jury on the fact that the defendant and certain physicians who were present in the court had not been called by the defendant as witnesses. The judge expressed his disapprobation of this line of remark, and instructed the jury, in his general charge, that they were to draw no presumptions from the fact that those persons were not called as witnesses. We are unable to perceive how the defendant could possibly be prejudiced by the remarks of counsel, thus promptly counteracted. Besides, it is quite probable that counsel had the right to make such comment. This disposes of all the exceptions upon which error is assigned adversely to the defendant. The judgment of the circuit court must be affirmed.

(B)
LEGAL DECISIONS AND COMMENTS

I.

The basis for chiropractic practice is the adjustment by hands of the spinal column.

1. Michigan, chiropractic law chapter 121a, section 14.596.
2. State v. Boston (1938), 226 Iowa 429, 278 N.W. 291, (re-hearing-284 N.W. 143).
3. State v. Grayson (1958), 5 Wis. 2d 203, 92 N.W. 2d 272.
4. People v. Fowler (1938), 32 CA 2d 737, 84 P 2d 326.
5. People v. Mangiagli (1950), 97 CA 2d 935, 218 P 2d 1025.

II.

The practice of chiropractic does not include the use of therapeutic adjuncts and modalities, nor vitamins or dietary supplements.

1. State v. Boston, supra.
2. State v. Grayson, supra.
3. Kuhl v. Arkansas State Board of Chiropractic Examiners, 364 S.W. 2d 790.
4. Arkansas Chiropractic Law Chapter - 72-404.

III.

The use of adjuncts and modalities in broad law states is to be restricted to supplemental assistance and necessity to the spinal adjusting.

1. State v. Fowler, supra.
2. State v. Mangiagli, supra.

IV.

Chiropractic restricted to a specific portion of the body is a proper subject for licensure separate from the medical profession.

1. Schlichting v. Texas State Board of Medical Examiners (1958-Naturopathy), 310 S.W. 2d 557.

2. Davis v. Beeler (1947-Naturopathy), 207 S.W. 2d 343.

3. Howe v. Smith (1964), 199 A. 2d 521.

4. See also Boston and Grayson cases, supra.

V.

A chiropractor is entitled to be judged by a standard of care based upon his education and community practice, so long as he does not treat or diagnose according to medical or other methods.

1. Correll v. Goodfellow, (1964) 125 N.W. 2d 745.

2. Attorney General Letter to Vice President of Chiropractic Examining Board of Tennessee (1964).

3. Attorney General Letter to Oregon Naturopathy Board of Examiners (1952).

4. See also Kuhl, Boston, Grayson, Fowler and Mangiagli cases, supra.

Discussion

Presently, 47 of the 50 United States recognize the profession of chiropractic by licensure. Only the states of Massachusetts, Mississippi, and Louisiana do not yet so recognize chiropractic. However, even in these states the practice is permitted although unregulated.* Additionally, about half of these states require that prospective chiropractors sit for the same Basic Science examinations as those given to the medical profession's candidates.

The Boston case cited above reached the Supreme Court of the state of Iowa in 1938. A chiropractor by the name of Boston had been practicing in the city of Davenport and allegedly had used physiotherapy, electrotherapy, colonic irrigations and diet. The Iowa court in holding against the chiropractor stated that the legislature intended to define and limit the field of chiropractic and that under the Iowa statute, a chiropractor was not authorized to practice physiotherapy, electrotherapy, colonic irrigation, or to prescribe diet for patients, **since such practices are outside the field to which the practice of chiropractic has been limited.***

----

* Author's Note: Chiropractic is now licensed in all of the 50 states of the United States."

* Author's Note: Chiropractic defined, Iowa House File 299, an act relating to the practice of chiropractic section 1. Section one hundred fifty-one point one (151.1) subsection two (2) code 1973, is amended by striking the subsection and inserting in lieu thereof the following: (2) persons who treat human ailments by the adjustment of the musculo skeletal structures, primarily spinal adjustments by hand, or by other procedures incidental to said adjustments limited to heat, cold, exercise, and supports the principals of which chiropractors are subject to examination under the provisions of section one hundred fifty-one point three (151.3) of the code, but not as independent therapeutic means.

The court went on to enjoin Dr. Boston from using physiotherapy, electrotherapy, colonic irrigation, colon hygiene, ultra-violet rays, infrared rays, radionics machines, traction tables, white lights, cold quartz ultraviolet light, neuroelectric vitalizer, electric vibrator, galvanic current and sinusoidal current for the purpose of treatment of the sick or for any other purpose in connection with his practice of chiropractic, and from the use of medicine and surgery and from prescribing certain or specific course of diet for any patient as an independent remedy or means of treatment.

An interesting point in this case is that the 1938 decision expressly did not enjoin the doctor from "using his reasonable judgment in recommending to a patient certain changes in diet, exercise or such of his general habits as affect his health...", but when the case came on for a rehearing in 1939, the court sustained the appeal of the state and enjoined the defendant further from advising as to diet. The court further quoted from legal works to show that the very word "chiropractic" meant that which is done by hand in upholding its decision against the use by chiropractors of other means and machinery.

The Grayson case cited above occurred in Wisconsin and the decision of the Supreme Court of that state was handed down in October of 1958. That decision enjoined the chiropractor from the use of a whole series of adjuncts and modalities, at least two of which have since been condemned by action of an administrative agency of the Health and Welfare Department of the federal government, the Food and Drug Administration.

The Wisconsin court upheld a rule of the Chiropractic

Board of Examiners of Wisconsin in ruling that the use of diagnostic instruments as taught in chiropractic colleges and generally used in chiropractic practice are permissible in the practice of chiropractic, but that use of instruments or machines, constituting specific therapies in themselves such as: colonic irrigators, diathermy, plasmatic, short wave, radionics, ultrasonic, and others, are considered outside the scope of chiropractic practice.

The above cases from Iowa and Wisconsin are authority for the proposition that the practice of chiropractic does not include the use of therapeutic adjuncts and modalities. Further, and very recently, the Arkansas Supreme Court in Kuhl v. Arkansas State Board of Chiropractic Examiners upheld the revocation of two chiropractors' licenses by that state's Board of Chiropractic Examiners when these doctors claimed to be qualified to dispense vitamins and supplements, do plasmatic therapy, traction, muscle stimulations, diathermy, ultrasonic therapy, infrared therapy, ear irrigations, x-rays and fluoroscopy, endo- or electrocardiograms, special interpretations, laboratory examinations, physical examinations, basal metabolism, hydrotherapy and blood counts and urine analysis.

The Arkansas court stated that the evidence that the chiropractors were engaged in the illegal practice of medicine was overwhelming and that the case was an aggravated one.

Even in states which have broad laws regarding licensure of chiropractors, the courts when requested have restricted the use of adjuncts and modalities to direct assistance and necessity to the spinal adjustments.

In the case of People v. Fowler, supra, the municipal court of Los Angeles had convicted the defendant of a misdemeanor for practicing a system and mode of treating the sick without having a valid unrevoked license authorizing him to do so. This was true even though the defendant was a licensed chiropractor. The Supreme Court of California affirmed the conviction.

The defendant cited the case of Evans v. McGranahan (1935), 4 Cal. App. 2d 202, 41 P. 2d 937, as support for his contention that section 7 of the California chiropractic act permitted him to do everything that was taught in chiropractic schools and colleges. The court stated that the defendant's interpretation of the law was too broad and went on to stress the wording of the statute in that the practice authorized must be chiropractic as taught in chiropractic schools and colleges. The court then went on to take pains to refer to dictionary and legal reference definitions pinpointing chiropractic as a system of vertebral adjustment.

The defendant further had contended that section 7 of the chiropractic act permitting him ''to use all necessary mechanical, and hygienic and sanitary measures incident to the care of the body'', was a definition of chiropractic. The court disagreed stating that this language was simply an addition to chiropractic in the state, and went on to stress that these allowances under the chiropractic law could not be used to invade the medical field.

The case of People v. Mangiagli, supra, was a case in which the defendant chiropractor was charged with the practice of medicine without an unrevoked certificate even though he was a licensed chiropractor. In this case the defendant had given blood plasma and a hypodermic injection. The court went on to approve and reconfirm the Fowler decision and stated that it was clear that the administration of blood plasma and the injection, when done for the treatment of ailment, disease, or other physical condition, are not such mechanical, hygienic or sanitary measures incident to the care of the body as may be used by chiropractic licensees.

Moreover, the attorney general from the state of Oregon in a letter written to the Naturopathic Board of Examiners on April 11, 1952, made it clear that holders of licenses to practice chiropractic and naturopathy are not to give injections. The opinion indicates that the giving of injections is the administration of drugs and is not permitted.

It is pointed out that chiropractic has come of age as a profession, even as it was necessary for the medical profession to come of age and eliminate many of its abuses and upgrade its educational standards. It is therefore fair to state that chiropractic restricted to a specific portion of the body is a proper subject for licensure separate and distinct from the medical profession, so long as it is maintained separate and distinct from the medical profession.

In this respect, the naturopathy cases in Tennessee and Texas, supra, in which licensure of naturopaths under separate licensing laws were held to be unconstitutional, or fit subjects for repeal, substantiate the above statement. Particularly, in the Texas case of Schlichting v. Texas State Board of Medical Examiners, supra, it is to be noted that the court carefully distinguished between the practice of naturopathy, which purported to care for the whole body as against those specific healing arts of chiropractic, dentistry, and optometry, which were limited to a specific portion of the body. The court stated that the practice of naturopathy was all right so long as the individuals practicing it first obtained a medical degree. The distinction was then made that the naturopath cared for the whole body as does the medical doctor and should not be licensed without first obtaining the necessary education and skills. It is therefore submitted that extension of the scope of practice to chiropractors of those things which are outside of their field would, in effect, place the profession in danger of extinction as a separate and distinct healing art.

Moreover, attention is directed to the case of Howe v. Smith, supra, which was a recent proceeding by chiropractors to enjoin the Secretary of Revenue in the state of Pennsylvania from refusing to accept certificates from chiropractors concerning physical fitness of motor vehicle operators. The Supreme Court affirmed the lower court decision against the chiropractors holding that the Secretary of Revenue who accepted physical examinations of motor vehicle operators by physicians but not examinations by chiropractors was exercising discretion given him by the legislature and was not unconstitutional discrimination between the two professions.

The case went on to point out that a limited license issued under the medical practice act permitting the licensing of chiropractors did not authorize the chiropractic licensee to practice medicine or the healing arts generally.

It is now generally understood that a chiropractor is entitled to be judged by his own standard of care where he is accused of malpractice, so long as he does not treat or diagnose according to medical or other methods. This was recently brought out in the Correll v. Goodfellow case, supra. In this case, the chiropractor had used an ultrasonic machine on the defendant's legs. The defendant happened to be diabetic and brought a case of malpractice for injury against the chiropractor. The lower court held for the chiropractor, but on appeal, the supreme court remanded the case for a new trial stating that in going outside the practice of chiropractic and entering the field of medicine by administering ultrasonic treatments, the chiropractor was held to the care and skill usually exercised by medical doctors.

In a 1964 letter to the vice president of the Tennessee State Board of Chiropractic Examiners, the attorney general of that state pointed out that the practice of chiropractic was limited to the science of palpating, analyzing, and adjusting the articulations of the human spinal column and adjacent tissues by hand. It was further stated in the letter that x-ray machines, electrical devices, etc., may be used by chiropractors only if they are necessarily incidental to the performance of this science. This would appear to follow the California case as cited above. Also, the Tennessee attorney general pointed out that since the chiropractor is not trained as a medical doctor he should not be permitted to take blood.

It is therefore submitted that a legislative broadening of the practice of chiropractic to include various therapies, etc., simply opens a "Pandora's box" of legal tribulation for years to come. Moreover, it is further submitted that by so broadening the practice, such action would endanger the maintenance of the chiropractic profession as a separate and distinct healing science.

We would be remiss also not to take the time to point out that insurers are willing to recognize chiropractic services in offering such to their policyholders, but not where violence is to be done to their premium rate structure when the chiropractic practitioner invades other healing arts through a duplication of service. In this respect, it should be noted certain of the Federal Benefit Plans have adopted specific language regarding chiropractic services. An example of such language is attached to this brief and made a part of it by reference.

Also, for convenience, we are attaching copies of some of the references which are used in this brief, insofar as it has been convenient to do so. Therefore, numbering them as exhibits beginning at Arabic numeral one and proceeding in progression, we attach copies of the following as exhibits with this brief and by reference and attachment make them a part hereof. These exhibits in order of their exhibit numbers are the Boston case, the Grayson case, the Kuhl case, the Schlichting case, the Davis case, the Howe case, and the Goodfellow case.

STATE V. BOSTON
Exhibit I
No. 43483.
(*Supreme Court of Iowa. March 15, 1938.*)

1. Physicians And Surgeons - 6 (1)

Under statute authorizing the practice of "chiropractic" to treat human ailments and defining "chiropractic," person using other modalities than those defined in statute as a curative means or methods was attempting to function outside the restricted field to which the practice of chiropractic has been limited. Code 1935, 2555.

2. Physicians And Surgeons - 6 (1)

Under statute authorizing the practice of chiropractic, defining the treatment, and providing that license to practice shall not authorize practice of operative surgery, osteopathy, nor the administration or prescription of any drug or medicines included in materia medica, Legislature intended to define and limit the field of chiropractic, and the maxim that the expressed controls or excludes the unmentioned was inapplicable. Code 1935, § 2559.

3. Physicians And Surgeons - 6 (1)

Under statute limiting field of chiropractic treatments of human ailments, a chiropractor was not authorized to practice physiotherapy, electrotherapy, colonic irrigation, or to prescribe diet for patients, since such practices are outside the field to which practice of chiropractic has been limited. Code 1935, § 2555.

HAMILTON, J., dissenting

Appeal from District Court, Scott County; Wm. W. Scott, Judge.

Equity action to restrain defendant by injunction from alleged unlawful practice of medicine. From the degree of the trial court, both parties appealed.

Reversed on plaintiff's appeal, with instructions.

Affirmed on defendant's appeal.

Block, Block & Agnew, of Davenport, and John Mitchell, Atty. Gen., for appellant.

A. T. Holmes, of LaCrosse, Wis. J. M. Maloney, of Davenport, L. E. Linnan, of Algona, and W. B. Sloan, of Des Moines, for appellee and cross-appellant.

RICHARDS, Justice.

During the period within which occurred the transactions hereinafter related, defendant held a license issued by the proper state authorities to practice chiropractic. At no time was he licensed to practice medicine and surgery. It is claimed by plaintiff that certain practices on part of defendant were unauthorized under the license he held and constituted unlawful practice of medicine and surgery. To restrain such practices by injunction this action in equity was instituted by the State of Iowa. The district court granted the full relief prayed by plaintiff, excepting that in enjoining defendant from one of these practices, that is, the prescribing of specific courses of diet, the court provided that the decree should not enjoin defendant "from using his reasonable judgment in recommending to a patient certain changes of diet, exercise or such of his general habits as affect his health." From the portion of the decree that appears above as a quotation plaintiff has appealed and claims with respect thereto that prescribing of diet should have been wholly enjoined. Afterwards defendant appealed from the decree as a whole.

Defendant held himself out, including the using of newspaper and telephone directory advertising, as practicing physiotherapy, electrotherapy, colonic irrigation, and diet. In some advertisements he designated himself as being a chiropractor and physiotherapist. In his office in Davenport where he treated patients defendant had a number of mechanical appliances, some of which brought electric and galvanic currents into contact with the patient's body. Rays emanating from other machines or appliances raised the temperature of portions of the patient's body, while another imparted a physical vibration to the part of the body with which it was contacted. There was a "colonic irrigator" wherewith about two gallons of water was used as an enema, the procedure lasting from 20 to 30 minutes. Defendant also advised patients with respect to diet. It is to these and other modalities that the decree of injunction applied. Later in this opinion a portion of the decree is set out.

(1) The question presented is whether the district court correctly held that the use of these things in the treatment of human ailments was not chiropractic, but constitutes practice of medicine. Section 2555, Code 1935, so far as pertinent to this case, is in these words:

"2555. Chiropractic defined. For the purpose of this title the following classes of persons shall be deemed to be engaged in the practice of chiropractic:

"1. * * *

"2. Persons who treat human ailments by the adjustment by hand of the articulations of the spine or by other incidental adjustments."

In this statute is found the only source of defendant's authority to treat human ailments. Likewise therein is a legislative definition of what such treating of human ailments consists, i.e., adjustment by hand of the articulations of the spine or other incidental adjustments. When defendant professed to use and used modalities other than those defined in section 2555, as curative means or methods, the conclusion seems unavoidable that he was attempting to function outside the restricted field of endeavor to which the Legislature has limited the practice of chiropractic. The only authority bearing on this question that has come to our attention is Heintze v. New Jersey State Board of Medical Examiners, 107 N.J.L. 420, 153 A. 253. In that case, Heintze, referred to in the opinion as prosecutor, had been convicted in the lower court of the penal offense of practicing medicine and surgery without having been licensed so to do. Prosecutor, Heintze, was a chiropractor. The opinion does not set out the New Jersey statutes defining the nature of the practice of chiropractic, but the defendant in the case at bar admits in argument that these statutes, chapter 4 of the Public Laws of 1920, afterwards repealed, defined the treatment of chiropractic as "by hand." We quote from the opinion in the cited case:

"The prosecutor is a chiropractor licensed under chapter 4 of the laws of 1920, which was later repealed, but saving licenses issued thereunder. He used the word 'Doctor' as a title; diagnosed; and treated patients, not only by manual manipulation within the act of 1920, but by the use of vibrator, electric light, galvanic current, etc. His female assistant, in his presence, gave directions for a vegetarian diet and the use of flaxseed tea. That such practice is outside of a license to use chiropractic, and within the domain of medicine and surgery, seems entirely plain. Clearly, therefore, the case was in one or more respects within the statute, prescribing a penalty for practicing without a medical license. It may well be that the use of the word 'Doctor' by a regularly licensed chiropractor is permissible; we do not rest on that; but the other practices just mentioned are not."

(2) Defendant draws from section 2559, Code 1935, certain inferences to support the proposition that as a

chiropractor he had the right to practice in the manner shown. Section 2559 provides that a license to practice chiropractic shall not authorize the licensee to practice operative surgery, osteopathy, nor administer or prescribe any drug or medicines included in materia medica. Relying on the maxim 'expressio unius est exclusio alterius,' defendant urges that, because in this statute the thing prohibited is administering or prescribing any drug or medicine included in materia medica a legislative intent is shown to authorize chiropractors to use medicine in the board general definition of a remedial agent or remedy. Defendant says that the statute did not add the words 'vibrator,' 'traction tables,' 'ultra-violet rays,' 'infrared lamps,' 'galvanic current,' to the prohibitory words of section 2559, and that it is obvious these words cannot be added except by Legislature.

The case of Bay v. Davidson, 133 Iowa 688, 111 N.W. 25, 27, 9 L.R.A., N.S., 1014, 119 Am.St.Rep. 650, throws some light upon the limitations incident to the application of the maxim on which defendant relies. The plaintiffs in that case, who were residents and taxpayers of the town of Grand River, sought to enjoin payment for materials and machines sold to the town by the defendants, who were the mayor and members of the town council. Because defendants were such officers it was claimed by plaintiffs that the sales were unlawful. At the time of the sales, section 668, Code 1897, provided that no members of any council shall be interested in any contract or job for work, or the profits thereof, or services to be performed for the corporation. Defendants contended that, as this statute put restraint upon only such contracts as have in view the performance of service or work, it was an abrogation of the common law rule that related to other contracts. Discussing this contention, the opinion says:

"This position is wholly untenable. It would seem that counsel have in mind the maxim 'expressio unius est exclusio alterius,' (the naming of one person or thing is an exclusion of the other). Reflection will make it clear that the maxim cannot be given application to work a result as here contended for. We have already said in this opinion that contracts of the character here in question are not included in the statute, and this, because the statute refers only to contracts for service or labor. And, in so holding, we have in a sense made application of the maxim above quoted. And, as we have seen, the decree was not predicated upon the statute, and there is no authority, as there can be no reason, for invoking the maxim to give validity to a contract void at common law as against public policy simply because it does not fall within the provisions of the statute. Both contracts for service and contracts of sale are prohibited at common law. The Legislature has done nothing more than to emphasize the prohibition as to service contracts. And, in our opinion, it would be absurd to give effect to the statute as evidencing at once a change of view respecting the matter of public policy, and as a declaration for the legality of all contracts theretofore within the class prohibited at common law save those in such statute prohibited in terms."

As already indicated, it appears to us that in section 2555 the Legislature intended to define and limit the field of chiropractic. This limitation being mentioned in a preceding section of the act, there would appear to be, as to section 2559, no clear necessity for application of the maxim that the expressed controls or excludes the unmentioned. For it may correctly be said that the limitation, being that which defendant would exclude by the maxim, is not something unmentioned. As in the cited cases, we are inclined to look upon section 2559 as doing nothing more than emphasize the prohibition as to materia medica. We think this ascribes to each section, without conflict between them, the true legislative intent. The injunctive portion of the decree of the trial court was as follows:

"Wherefore it is ordered, adjudged and decreed that the defendant, Charles J. Boston, be and he hereby is forever enjoined from the use of physiotherapy, electrotherapy, colonic irrigation, colon hygiene, ultra-violet rays, infrared rays, radionics machines, traction tables, white lights, cold quartz ultra-violet light, neurolectric vitalizer, electric vibrator, galvanic current and sinusoidal current for the purpose of treatment of the sick or for any other purpose in connection with his practice of chiropractic and from the use of medicine and surgery and from prescribing certain or specific course of diet for any patient as an independent remedy or means of treatment. Defendant is not enjoined from using his reasonable judgment in recommending to a patient certain changes in diet, exercise or such of his general habits as affect his health but is enjoined from prescribing any specific or certain course of diet as above set out.

"The defendant is further enjoined from advertising his use of physiotherapy, electrotherapy, colonic irrigation, colon hygiene, ultra-violet rays, infrared rays, radionics machines, traction tables, white lights, cold quartz ultra-violet light, neurolectric vitalizer, electric vibrator, galvanic current and sinusoidal current or any of them in the treatment of the sick or as an aid to or preliminary or preparatory to his use of chiropractic or in any other way holding out to the public that any of these means or modalities may be or are used by him in the treatment of the sick or as an aid to or preliminary or preparatory to the use of chiropractic or for any other purpose and from assuming or publicly professing to assume the duties of a physician and surgeon or from using mechanical or electrical means or modalities in the practice of chiropractic or as an aid to or preliminary or preparatory to the use of chiropractic or from using to publicly professing to use any mode or general course of treatment other than chiropractic adjustments, and the Clerk is hereby ordered to issue an injunction in accordance with this decree."

We approve the decree as restraining defendant from professing to and treating human ailments in modes and manners outside the field of chiropractic, excepting that defendant should have been enjoined wholly from the prescribing for or the advising of his patients with respect to diet. The case is affirmed on defendant's appeal and reversed on plaintiff's appeal, with directions that a decree be entered in the district court in conformity herewith.

Affirmed on defendant's appeal.

Reversed on plaintiff's appeal, with instructions.

SAGER, ANDERSON, KINTIZINGER, AND MILLER, JJ., concur.

HAMILTON, J. dissenting, would affirm on both appeals.

STATE V. BOSTON
No. 43483
(Supreme Court of Iowa. Feb. 15, 1939.)

1. Physicians And Surgeons - 6 (1)

The practice of "medicine and surgery" is the practice of the healing art, and unless some restriction is placed thereon by the legislature, the whole field of medicine and surgery is open to the practitioner.

Ed. Note.—For other definitions of "Medicine or Surgery," see Words & Phrases.

2. Physicians And Surgeons - 6 (1)

A statute providing that a license to practice chiropractic did not authorize licensees to do certain things did not authorize licensee to do all of the things not therein prohibited, where another statute defined the practice of chiropractic. Code 1935, § 2555, 2559.

Appeal from District Court, Scott County; Wm. W. Scott, Judge.

Equity action to restrain defendant by injunction from alleged unlawful practice of medicine. From the decree of the trial court both parties appealed.

Reversed on plaintiff's appeal, with instructions. Affirmed on defendant's appeal.

Supplementing opinion in 278 N.W. 291.

John J. Mitchell, Atty. Gen., and Block, Block & Agnew of Davenport, for the State.

A. T. Holmes of LaCrosse, Wis., J. M. Maloney, of Davenport, L. E. Linnan, of Algona, and W. B. Sloan, of Des Moines, for appellee.

HALE, Justice.

The facts are fully set out in the former opinion, reported in 278 N.W. 291, of which this supplemental opinion is now made a part.

The injunctive portion of the decree of the trial court is set out in the original opinion and only needs to be referred to here. In short, it forbids the use of certain appliances or modalities, but permits defendant to recommend to a patient changes in diet, under certain restrictions. From the decree, except as to that part concerning diet, defendant appealed; and from that part permitting advising as to diet, the State appealed. The appeal was heard and determined in this court, and was reversed on plaintiff's appeal, with instruction, and affirmed on defendant's appeal. State v. Boston, 278, N.W. 291, 292.

Rehearing was granted June 24, 1938, and the case is now before us on such rehearing.

The defendant in his reply to plaintiff's argument on rehearing alleges that there is only one issue in this case, and that is: "Do the things which the evidence shows the defendant did, constitute the practice of medicine and surgery?" Such was the question on the former hearing: "Whether the district court correctly held that the use of these things in the treatment of human ailments was not chiropractic, but constitutes practice of medicine."

This case was thoroughly argued and presented on the former hearing, and in the argument on this rehearing little has been added other than to amplify the arguments on the former submission. The defendant urges, as on the former hearing, that the statutes of Iowa make a chiropractor a member of the healing professions, with authority to use any agency in accomplishing this result of healing the sick so long as he did not violate the express statutory provisions found in the Code; and that our interpretation of the statutes permitting and regulating the practice of his profession is too narrow in restricting the persons so practicing to the provisions of section 2555 of the Code.

We repeat the provisions of that section, so far as applicable: "Persons who treat human ailments by the adjustment by hand of the articulations of the spine or by other incidental adjustments."

The statutory definition does not vary to any great extent from the well-known and generally accepted definition of this form of the healing art.

See II C. J. p. 758: "Chiropractics. A system of healing that treats disease by manipulation of the spinal column; the specific science that removes pressure on the nerves by the adjustment of the spinal vertebrae. There are no instruments used, the treatment being by hand only. The word is coined from two Greek words 'chiro' and 'practicas,' signifying something done with the hands." (Cases cited.)

Ballantine's Law Dictionary defines "chiropractic" as follows: "The word is derived from the Greek, and means, primarily, to do by hand,—hand manipulation. Webster's New International Dictionary defines chiropractic to be a system of healing that treats disease by manipulation of the spinal column."

(1, 2) The practice of medicine and surgery is the practice of the healing art, and, unless some restriction be placed thereon by the legislature, the whole field of medicine and surgery is open to the practitioner. On the other hand, the practice of chiropractic, although recognized as a branch of the healing art, is throughout held and considered to be only one form of the practice, within well-defined limits, of the science of healing, as such practice is defined by Code, § 2555. That is the method which may be used. To this the legislature has added, in section 2559, certain prohibitions. The legislature has prescribed the method of healing which may be used by these practitioners, and has further mentioned other methods which may not be used. The original opinion, describing the method these practitioners may employ, holds that these restrictions merely emphasize the limitations laid down in section 2555, to which defendant takes exception.

If section 2559 broadened the field in which the chiropractor might practice, and if he has the right to go outside the restrictions and employ other methods except such as are therein prohibited, then the whole field of medical science is open to him except as prohibited in that section. This defendant cannot claim. We believe that medicine and surgery comprehend the whole field of medicine and materia medica; and that it was the intent of the legislature that chiropractic should be merely a form of treatment, and that it must be practiced according to the rules laid down by law. Whether or not the limitations are proper or too restrictive is not for this court to say.

If the use of these modalities is forbidden to the chiropractor, but they are used in the practice of medicine and surgery, as is held in the former opinion, to which we adhere, then this action was properly brought for a violation of the medical practice act.

It seems to us that the use of the appliances or modalities in the case at bar does come within the domain of medicine and surgery and would constitute a part of that practice. Therefore, as it constitutes a part of the practice of medicine and surgery, and does not come within the definition of chiropractic, the injunction was properly issued.

It is urged that adherence to our former opinion will bar the use of mechanical appliances or common instruments by barbers, coaches, and others. The classes mentioned are not engaged in the practice of medicine, or of healing, nor are they holding themselves out to the public as healers.

The reason for all laws restricting this and other professions is the protection of the public, and to that end the legislature has seen fit to enact laws and provide means for enforcing the regulations governing the practice of the various forms of the art of healing, permitting each practitioner to follow his profession according to its established principles. Each may have its merits; but those persons who are authorized to practice one form of the art may not encroach upon another form for which they have not authority from the state.

The case is affirmed on defendant's appeal and reversed on plaintiff's appeal, with directions that a decree be entered in conformity herewith.—Reversed on plaintiff's appeal, with instructions. Affirmed on defendant's appeal.

RICHARDS, SAGER, MILLER, AND OLIVER, JJ., concur.

(5 Wis. 2d 203)
STATE OF WISCONSIN, RESPONDENT, EXHIBIT II
v.
ROBERT L. GRAYSON, APPELLANT
(*Supreme Court of Wisconsin. Oct. 7, 1958.*)

The State of Wisconsin brought action against chiropractor to enjoin him from treating the sick by use of allegedly unauthorized procedures, machines, and instruments and from using the title of "Dr.," "Doctor," or "D.C." the Circuit Court for Kenoshal County, M. Eugene Baker, J., entered an order sustaining the demurrer of the State to certain paragraphs of the answer, and the chiropractor appealed. The Supreme Court, Currie, J., held that definition of "chiropractic" by Chiropractic Board of Examiners as science based on premise that disease or abnormal function is caused by interference with normal nerve transmission and expression, due primarily to pressure, strain, irritation, or tension on spinal nerves as they emit from spinal column, as result of bony segments, especially of the spine, deviating from their normal juxtaposition, and that practice of "chiropractic" consists of analysis of any interference with normal nerve transmission and expression and correction thereof by specific adjustment with the hands of abnormal deviations of bony articulations especially of the spine, for removal of cause of disease, without use of drugs or surgery, is a valid rule.

Order affirmed

1. Physicians And Surgeons - 6 (1)

Chiropractors, who are licensed under statute, are authorized to treat the sick only to extent authorized by their chiropractic licenses. W.S.A. 147.14, 147.23

2. Physicians And Surgeons - 6 (1)

Where the Legislature, in enacting statute providing for the licensing of chiropractors, failed to define the term "chiropractic," it was for the Chiropractic Board of Examiners under provision of the Administrative Procedure Act that each agency is authorized to adopt such rules interpreting provisions of statutes enforced or administered by it as considers to be necessary to effectuate the purpose of the statutes, to define the term "chiropractic," and it was not for the courts to do so, and definition of the Chiropractic Board of Examiners was valid, if it did not exceed the bounds of correct interpretation. W.S.A. 147.23, 227.014 (2) (a).

3. Physicians And Surgeons - 6 (1)

Definition of "chiropractic" by Chiropractic Board of Examiners as science based on premise that disease or abnormal function is caused by interference with normal nerve transmission and expression, due primarily to pressure, strain, irritation, or tension on spinal nerves as they emit from spinal column, as result of bony segments, especially of the spine, deviating from their normal juxtaposition, and that practice of "chiropractic" consists of analysis of any interference with normal nerve transmission and expression and correction thereof by specific adjustment with the hands of abnormal deviations of bony articulations, especially of the spine, for removal of cause of disease, without use of drugs or surgery, is a valid rule. W.S.A. 147.23, 227.014 (2) (a).

See publication Words and Phrases, for other judicial constructions and definitions of "Chiropractic".

4. Physicians And Surgeons - 6 (1)

Rule of Chiropractic Board of Examiners that use of diagnostic instruments as taught in chiropractic colleges and generally used in chiropractic practice, as well as purely relaxing adjunct such as heat lamps or hot towels, used preparatory to adjustment, are permissible in practice of "chiropractic," but that use of instruments or machines, constituting specific therapies in themselves, such as colonic irrigators, diathermy, plasmatic, short-wave, radionics, ultrasonic, and others are considered outside the scope of chiropractic practice, is a valid rule. W.S.A. 147.23, 227.014 (2) (a).

5. Physicians And Surgeons - 6 (1)

Rule of the Chiropractic Board of Examiners that x-ray may be used for diagnostic or analytical purposes only is a valid rule. W.S.A. 147.23, 227.014, (2) (a).

6. Physicians And Surgeons - 6 (1)

Proviso in the Physical Therapy Licensing Statute that nothing in the statute shall be construed to restrict, inhibit, or limit practice of chiropractic as presently practiced in the state, and as taught by accredited schools or colleges of chiropractic is not an indication that chiropractors may practice physical therapy. W.S.A. 147.185.

Action instituted in the name of the state by the Attorney General to enjoin the defendant, who is a licensed chiropractor, from treating the sick by use of unauthorized procedures, machines, and instruments, and from use of the title "Dr.", "Doctor", or "D.C.".

Paragraph 17 of the complaint alleges that the defendant is engaged in the treatment of the sick by such unauthorized methods as:

"a. Punctures the skin and takes blood samples by use of an instrument described as a 'Spencer Hemogolobinometer,' which employs a spring operated lancet;

"b. Prescribes, suggests and advises course of diet and alleged corrective dietary habits;

"c. Prescribes, suggests, advises and dispenses food supplements and vitamins;

"d. Renders alleged psychosomatic counseling to his patients;

"e. Uses an instrument described as a De Wells 'Detoxicolon Therapy,' which purportedly introduces water containing organic mineral solution infused with oxygen into the intestinal tract;

"f. Uses an instrument described as a 'Plasmatic' machine, which purportedly produces heat electrically to raise body temperature;

"g. Uses an instrument described as a 'Raylax' table, which is represented as producing vibration, gravity, traction, and 'systemic' or 'local' heat therapy;

"h. Uses an instrument described as a 'myofasciatron Low Voltage Generator,' which produces a sinusoidal and galvanic current;

"i. Uses an instrument described as a 'Landum' lamp, which purportedly emits ultraviolet light for the alleged purpose of administering Vitamin D by radiation;

"j. Uses x-ray;

"k. Uses an instrument known as a 'Heart-ometer' represented as a method of determining blood vascular tone, heart strength amplitude and the like;

"l. Uses an instrument described as a 'Vitamoter Percussion' instrument represented as a mechanical massage instrument;

"m. Uses an instrument described as an 'Oster' represented as a massage instrument;

"n. Uses an instrument described as an 'Electrosonic' instrument represented as producing high frequency sound waves for therapeutic purposes;

"o. Uses an instrument described as 'Micro-Dynameter' represented as a method to measure the so-called 'Health Index,' and nerve function for diagnostic purposes to locate the point of interference on the spine, viscera and adjacent tissue."

The answer of the defendant admits that he employs all of the afore described methods in treating the sick except that he alleges he advises courses of diet and the use of food supplements and vitamins but does not prescribe the same. Certain affirmative defenses are alleged in such answer as follows:

"6. Alleges that the practice of chiropractic consists of the diagnosing of human ailments by the use of all diagnostic procedures recognized by the various schools of healing arts; the elimination of the abnormal functioning of the human nervous system by the adjustment of the articulations and adjacent tissue of the human body, particularly of the spinal column; the use, as indicated, of procedures which make the adjustment more effective, including clinical nutrition, psychotherapy and physiotherapy, but excluding the use of drugs and surgery.

"10. Alleges that for many years prior to the enactment of ch. 408 of the Wisconsin Laws of 1925 the practice of chiropractic included the use of such supplementary procedures as would increase the efficiency of the chiropractic adjustment as is more particularly set forth in paragraph 6 hereof, and that such use was well established in the profession and had substantial public acceptance.

"11. Alleges that the science and art of chiropractic has progressed and developed since the year 1925 and that from time to time new procedures have been developed and have gained acceptance by the profession and by the public generally.

"12. Alleges that eminent authority in the United States now accepts the practice of chiropractic as including procedures complementary to the chiropractic adjustment.

"13. Alleges that the determination of the scope of chiropractic practice in Wisconsin is a matter of public policy and beyond the authorization of this court to determine.

"14. Alleges that none of the instruments or procedures described in paragraph 17 of the complaint are detrimental to the health or well being of defendant's patients or the public in general."

The state demurred to each of the afore quoted paragraphs of the answers on the ground that each fails to state a defense. By order entered February 26, 1958, the trial court sustained the demurrer as to each of the attacked paragraphs. The defendant has appealed from such order.

Lucien J. Piery, Kenosha, Johns, Roraff, Pappas & Flaherty, La Crosse, for appellant.

Stewart G. Honeck, Atty. Gen., John D. Winner, Deputy Atty. Gen., John H. Bowers, Asst. Atty. Gen., for respondent.

CURRIE, Justice.

(1) Sec. 147.14, Stats., prohibits any person from treating the sick who does not hold a license or certificate of registration from the state board of medical examiners, "except as otherwise specifically provided by statute." By sec. 147.23 Stats., the legislature has provided for the licensing of chiropractors. It thereby necessarily follows that chiropractors so licensed are authorized to treat the sick only to the extent authorized by their chiropractic license.

To properly resolve the issue, of whether the paragraphs of the answer attacked by demurrer are irrelevant, requires that we make an analysis of the material provisions of sec. 147.23, Stats., and determine the validity of certain rules adopted by the chiropractic board of examiners in order to effectuate the purpose of such statute.

The procedure for licensing chiropractors embodied in sec. 147.23 was enacted by the 1925 legislature as ch. 408, Laws of 1925. This legislation originated in the assembly as Bill 322A. As originally introduced, such bill provided for a definition of "chiropractic" to be incorporated in the new statute as sub. (1) of sec. 147.23, Stats., reading as follows:

Chiropractic is defined as the adjustment by hand of

the articulation of the human vertebral column and the accessory articulation thereof." In enacting the bill the legislature amended the same by striking out such definition. The result is that sec. 147.23 has never contained a definition of the work "chiropractic."

Sub. (1) of sec. 147.23 provides that no person shall practice chiropractic unless he has a certificate of registration in the basic sciences and a license from the state board of examiners in chiropractic. Sub. (2) provides for the appointment of the three members of such licensing board of examiners by the governor with the consent of the senate, and states the necessary qualifications, compensation, and term of office of such board members.

Sub. (3) of such statutes establishes the necessary qualifications a person must possess in order to apply for a license in chiropractic. These are: good moral character, two years of study in a regularly prescribed course for a bachelor of arts or science degree in a college accredited by the North Central Association of Colleges and Secondary Schools, and graduation from a "reputable school of chiropractic" approved and recognized by the chiropractic board of examiners. Such school in chiropractic must be one having a residence course of 36 months consisting of not less than 3,600 sixty minute class periods.

Sub. (4) of such statute provides that the examination of applicants for a license shall be "in the subjects usually taught in such reputable schools of chiropractic."

Sec. 147.23 confers no express rule-making power upon the chiropractic board of examiners. However, sec. 227.014 (2) (a), which is part of the Wisconsin Administrative Procedure Act, does confer such power and provides:

"Each agency is authorized to adopt such rules interpreting the provisions of statutes enforced or administered by it as it considers to be necessary to effectuate the purpose of the statutes, but such rules are not valid if they exceed the bounds of correct interpretation."

The chiropractic board of examiners has adopted certain rules which have been duly published in the Wisconsin Administrative Code. We deem that of these rules, secs. Chir. 1.14, 3.01, and 3.02(1) are material to the issue before us on this appeal. We quote such rules as follows:

Chir. 1.14. "**Chiropractic defined.** The science of chiropractic is based upon the premise that disease or abnormal function is caused by interference with normal nerve transmission and expression, due primarily to pressure, strain, irritation or tension upon the spinal nerves as they emit from the spinal column, as a result of bony segments, especially of the spine, deviating from their normal juxtaposition. The practice of chiropractic consists of the analysis of any interference with normal nerve transmission and expression and the correction thereof by a specific adjustment with the hands of the abnormal deviations of the bony articulations, especially of the spine, for the removal of the cause of disease, without the use of drugs or surgery. The term, analysis, is construed to include the use of x-ray and other analytical instruments generally used in the practice of chiropractic."

Chir. 3.01 "**Supplementary procedures.** (1) The use of diagnostic instruments as taught in the chiropractic colleges and generally used in chiropractic practice, as well as purely relaxing adjuncts such as heat lamps or hot towels, used preparatory to the adjustment, are permissible. The use of instruments or machines constituting specific therapies in themselves, such as: Colonic irrigators, diathermy, plasmatic, short wave, radionics (various makes or versions), ultrasonic and others, are considered outside the scope of chiropractic practice in Wisconsin. (The foregoing are illustrative only and are not meant to be all inclusive).

"(2) Supplementary foods may be supplied for nutritional purposes in the original container, but may not be dispensed nor prescribed for specific conditions."

Chir. 3.02. "**X-ray.** (1) X-ray may be used for diagnostic or analytical purposes only."

If the afore quoted rules are valid, it readily appears that most of the methods and instrumentalities employed by the defendant, which are described in paragraph 17 of the compliant, are beyond the scope of the defendant's chiropractic license. Furthermore, if the validity of the rules is upheld, none of the attacked paragraphs of defendant's answer would constitute a defense and the trial court properly sustained the demurrer thereto.

The attorney general's brief quotes definitions of "chiropractic" to be found in various standard dictionaries and encyclopedias, which definitions are of the same restrictive character as that adopted by the licensing board in sec. Chir. 1.14. On the other hand, counsel for the defendant have provided the court with more liberal definitions of "chiropractic" set forth in the statutes of some of the other states. It also appears from the facts stated in the briefs that chiropractic colleges, and the chiropractors themselves, are in disagreement as to whether the practice of chiropractic is restricted to spinal adjustments made by the hands alone, or whether it includes certain adjunctive and complementary procedures, such as those employed by the defendant. It is conceded some of the chiropractic colleges do teach such supplementary methods of treatment.

The learned trial court in its memorandum opinion considered the issue presented by the demurrer as one which required the court to define the term "chiropractic." The trial court gave due consideration to the dictionary and encyclopedia definitions contained in the attorney general's brief, and, based upon such definitions, came to the following conclusion: "From these definitions and others it seems clear that the word ('chiropractic') is used to describe a system of treating the sick through the manipulation by hand of the spinal column."

The attorney general urges on this appeal that the trial court was correct in holding that it is the function of the courts to define "chiropractic" in the absence of the legislature doing so. On the other hand, counsel for the defendant contend that the courts are without power to define such term, and argue that the legislature intended that whatever practices the chiropractors engage in, and which the chiropractic colleges teach, should govern the scope of a state chiropractic license.

(2) It is our considered judgment that neither position is tenable. This is because the legislature has lodged the function of defining "chiropractic" with a state adminis-

trative agency, the chiropractic board of examiners, by sec. 227.014 (2) (a), Stats. It is difficult for us to conceive of any rule more necessary for such board to adopt, in effectuating the purpose of the chiropractic licensing statute, than one which defines the term "chiropractic." The validity of such definition embodied in the rule, which such board promulgated as one. Chir. 1.14 of the Wisconsin Administrative Code, is dependent upon whether it "exceeds the bounds of correct interpretation."

In People v. Fowler, 1938, 32 Cal. App. 2d Supp. 737, 84 P.2d 326, a California intermediate appellate court was called upon to determine the meaning of the word "chiropractic" in a California statute which did not define the term. It does not appear from the opinion therein that the legislature had delegated such power of definition to a licensing board or other state agency. The court arrived at a definition very similar in scope to that adopted by the Wisconsin Chiropratic board of examiners. Such definition was adhered to in the later case of People v. Mangiagli, 1950, 97 Cal. App. 2d Supp. 935, 218 P.2d 1025. The definition in sec. Chir. 1.14 is also fully consistent with the definitions of "Chiropractic" found in Funk and Wagnalls New Standard Dictionary of the English Language (Medallion ed. 1941) 469; Webster's New International Dictionary (2d Unabridged, 1935) 470; and 6 The Encyclopedia American (1945 ed.), 567-569. Furthermore, it is conceded that a considerable segment of the chiropractic profession and colleges champion this concept of chiropractic practice. We can perceive no clear cut legislative intent that the licensing board must adopt a definition so broad in scope as to permit every practice or procedure that may be taught in any chiropractic college.

(3-5) We, therefore, have no difficulty in determining that the definition of "chiropractic" set forth in sec. Chir. 1.14 does not exceed the bounds of correct interpretation and that such section constitutes a valid rule. Likewise, secs. Chir. 3.01 and 3.02(1), being entirely consistent with the definition set forth in sec. Chir. 1.14, are also a valid exercise by the licensing board of its rule-making power. These rules render the allegations of the answer, which were demurred to entirely irrelevant.

(6) One additional argument advanced in behalf of the defendant is deserving of comment. This is a contention that, when the legislature in 1953 enacted the physical therapy licensing statute (sec. 147.185, Stats.), it inserted a proviso therein which clearly indicated that chiropractors might practice physical therapy. From this it is further argued that the legislature thus manifested an intention that permissible chiropractic practice in Wisconsin is broader in scope than permitted by the above considered rules of the licensing board. We cannot agree with either the premise or the conclusion. The proviso thus alluded to constitutes sub. (7) of sec. 147.185, which provides as follows:

"Nothing in this section shall be construed to restrict, inhibit or limit the practice of chiropractic as now practiced in Wisconsin, and as taught by accredited schools or colleges of chiropractic."

Under Chir. Sec. 3.01 the use of heat lamps by licensed chiropractors as relaxing adjuncts preparatory to the spinal adjustment is permissible. The definition of the "practice of physical therapy" found in sub. (1) of sec.

147.185, is broad enough to include such use of heat
lamps. The legislature may well have concluded that the
proviso contained in sub. (7) of sec. 147.185 was necessary to remove any uncertainty as to the right of chiropractors to employ such heat lamps for the purpose
stated in sec. Chir. 3.01. We cannot construe sub. (7) of
sec. 147.185 as a grant of power in itself.

Order affirmed.

MARTIN, C. J. not participating.

WILLIAM E. KUHL AND ROBERT J. KUHL, EXHIBIT III APPELLANTS

v.

ARKANSAS STATE BOARD OF CHIROPRACTIC EXAMINERS, APPELLEE

No. 5-2874

(*Supreme Court of Arkansas. Feb. 4, 1963.*)

(*Rehearing Denied March 11, 1963.*)

Proceeding for revocation of chiropractors' licenses.
The State Board of Chiropractic Examiners revoked the
licenses, and the chiropractors brought certiorari. The
Circuit Court, Second Division, Pulaski County, Guy
Amsler, J., affirmed, and the chiropractors appealed. The
Supreme Court, Robinson, J., held that two chiropractors
who sent out literature offering to do laboratory work for
other chiropractors and stating that the other chiropractors might legally give medication for stomach worms or
pin-worms, and who sent out forms indicating that the
two chiropractors could diagnose many diseases, including cancer, by examining urine, illegally engaged in prac-

tice of medicine and did not confine themselves to practice of chiropractic.

Affirmed.

1. Physicians And Surgeons - 11 (3)

State Board of Chiropractic Examiners which filed charges alleging that chiropractors had illegally engaged in practice of medicine as charged in State Medical Board's complaint filed more than six months earlier did not err in overruling motion, which was not filed until day of hearing and under which chiropractors sought to have the charges made more definite and certain after having requested only immediate hearing.

2. Discover - 89

Action taken by State Board of Chiropractic Examiners in cases other than that involving two chiropractors charged with illegal practice of medicine would not have been relevant to chiropractors' case, and chiropractors were not entitled to delivery of all books, records, correspondence and minutes pertaining to disciplinary action taken or contemplated against any chiropractors since Board was created.

3. Physicians And Surgeons - 11 (3)

Error of member of State Board of Chiropractic Examiners in calling a doctor and questioning him about certain facts to determine if one of chiropractors charged with illegal practice of medicine had testified truthfully or falsely concerning his dealings with the hospital and treatment of hospital patients was harmless in view of other competent evidence showing that revocation of chiropractors' licenses was required.

4. Physicians And Surgeons - 11 (3)

State Board of Chiropractic Examiners is not bound by strict rules of evidence but the essential rules of evidence by which rights are asserted or defended must be preserved; however, hearing does not cease to be fair merely because rules of evidence and procedure applicable to judicial proceedings have not been strictly followed or evidence has been improperly rejected or received; to render hearing unfair, defect or practice must have been such as might have led to denial of justice, or element of due process must have been absent.

5. Physicians And Surgeons - 6 (1)

Two chiropractors who sent out literature offering to do laboratory work for other chiropractors and stating that the other chiropractors might legally give medication for stomach worms or pin-worms, and who sent out forms indicating that they could diagnose many diseases, including cancer, by examining urine, illegally engaged in practice of medicine and did not confine themselves to practice of chiropractic. Ark. Stats. §§ 72-404, 72-604

6. Physicians And Surgeons - 11 (3)

Authority of State Board of Chiropractic Examiners to revoke license of a chiropractor must be exercised in a proper manner and is not arbitrary. Ark. Stats.§ 72-407.

Dan McCraw, N. Little Rock, for appellants.

Martin, Dodds & Kidd, Little Rock, for Appellee.

ROBINSON, Justice.

The appellants, William E. and Robert J. Kuhl, are chiropractors authorized to practice in the State of Arkansas. On the 8th day of November, 1960, the Arkansas State Medical Board filed a complaint in the Pulaski

Chancery Court, wherein it was alleged that the above named appellants were engaged in the illegal practice of medicine in this state. The complaint alleged that the appellants were doing about a dozen different things that constituted the practice of medicine.[1]

On the 5th day of June, 1961, the Arkansas State Board of Chiropractic Examiners, acting on authority of Ark. Stats.§ 72-407, filed charges against appellants alleging that they had illegally engaged in the practice of medicine as charged in the complaint which had been filed in the Chancery Court by the Medical Board; and further, that they were guilty of unethical conduct. A summons was issued and served.

On June 13, 1961, appellants filed a motion asking that they be given an immediate hearing on the charges which had been filed on June 5. The hearing was set for June 28. On that date when the matter came on to be heard on the merits, appellants made an oral motion that the Chiropractic Board be required to make the charges more definite and certain. The motion was overruled and the Board proceeded with the hearing. After hearing all the evidence produced, the Chiropractic board ordered that appellants' license as chiropractors be revoked. By certiorari appellants took the case to Circuit Court where the order of the Board was affirmed.

(1) On appeal to this court appellants contend, first, that the Board's action in overruling the motion that the charges be made more definite and certain was error that calls for a reversal.

1. See Miller v. Reed, 234 Ark. 850, 355 S.W.2d, 169. We do not agree. The charges were filed by the Board and summons issued and served on June 5, 1961.

Allegations charging appellants with the illegal practice of medicine had been filed in Chancery Court by the Medical Board November 18, 1960, more than six months before the charges were filed by the Chiropractic Board. Moreover, during the interim between June 5, 1961 and the time of the hearing on June 28, the only thing filed by appellants was a request for an immediate hearing. Nor until the day of the hearing on June 28, did appellants ask that the charges be made more definite and certain. In these circumstances there was no error in denying the motion.

(2) While the matter was pending in the Circuit Court appellants filed a motion asking that the Chiropractic Board be required to deliver to the attorneys for appellants "all books, records, correspondence and minutes pertaining to any disciplinary action taken or contemplated against any chiropractor since the creation of the board for the purpose of permitting defendants to inspect same and copy if desired." The motion was overruled by the trial court. We fail to see in what manner the action taken by the Board in some other case would be relevant to the case at bar.

(3) After the taking of testimony before the Chiropractic Board and while the matter was still in the hands of the Board, Dr. Murphy, a member of the Board, called a doctor on the staff of the Missouri Pacific Hospital and questioned him about certain facts to determine if appellant, Dr. William Kuhl, had testified truthfully or falsely concerning his dealings with the hospital and the treatment of Missouri Pacific Hospital patients. Of course, if the judge of a court or a juror adopted such means to ascertain the facts, we would quickly hold that it was error to obtain evidence in that fashion. But members of the Chiropractic Board are not lawyers and they are not

jurors with a judge available to tell them what they may or may not do. In all probability, members of the Chiropractic Board know nothing about the rules of evidence and perhaps they could never hear an involved case without making errors in admitting or rejecting evidence, if their action in that respect were tested by the rules of evidence applicable to a court of law.

In Bockman v. Arkansas State Medical Board, 229 Ark. 143, 313 S.W. 2d 826, we had the same point under consideration and there we said: "This is not a criminal prosecution, in which the accused is entitled to be confronted by the witnesses against him. It is an administrative proceeding, civil in nature,..." It is further stated in that case that the Board could not proceed at all if it were required to observe technical rules of evidence. Also we said in the Bockman case: "Upon this point it is our rule in proceedings like this one that the board's action will not be set aside on certiorari unless there is an entire absence of substantial evidence to sustain the findings,...". But even so, we would send this case back to the Board of Chiropractic Examiners for a new trial if it appeared that appellants did not receive a fair trial, or that Dr. Murphy's action in talking to a doctor at the Missouri Pacific Hospital, and perhaps other chiropractors, was in an any way prejudicial to appellants; but we cannot see how appellants were prejudiced in any manner by the conversations, because regardless of what was said, and notwithstanding anything that may have been said, there is competent evidence in the record which shows that appellants' license to practice chiropractic must be revoked.

(4) Even though the Board is not bound by strict rules

of evidence, the essential rules of evidence by which rights are asserted or defended must be preserved. But a hearing does not cease to be fair merely because rules of evidence and procedure applicable in judicial proceedings have not been strictly followed, or because some evidence has been improperly rejected or received. Bilokumsky v. Tod, 263 U.S. 149, 44 S. Ct.54, 68 L.Ed. 221. To render a hearing unfair, the defect or practice must have been such as might have led to a denial of justice, or there must have been absent one of the elements of due process.

Ark. Stats. § 72-604 defines the practice of medicine, in part as follows: "...suggesting, recommending, prescribing or administering any form of treatment, operation or healing for the intended palliation, relief, or cure of any physical or mental disease, ailment, injury, condition or defect of any person with the intention of receivng therefore, either directly or indirectly, any fee, gift, or compensation whatsoever,..."

A chiropractic license entitles "the holder, thereof to adjust by hand the displaced segments of the vertebral column and any displaced tissue in any manner related thereto for the purpose of removing any injury, deformity or abnormality of human beings," Ark. Stats. §72-404.

(5) Of course, if any information Dr. Murphy obtained not in the presence of appellants, had to be relied on in any respect to support a finding that appellants, unlawfully engaged in the practice of medicine, the judgment would have to be reversed; but such is not the case. The printed matter on appellants' statement of account form contains a list of the treatments they hold themselves out as giving, which are listed as follows:

"(1) Adjustments, (2) Vitamins or Supplements, (3) Plasmatic Therapy, (4) Traction, (5) Muscle Stimulation, (6) Diathermy, The generation of heat in tissues of the body, as a result of the resistance presented by the tissue to electric currents of high frequency that is forced through them. (7) Ultrasonic Therapy, Super sound wave treatment, (8) Infrared Therapy, Pertaining to or designating those rays which lie just beyond the red end of the visible spectrum, such as are emitted by a hot nonincandescent body. They are invisible and non-actinic and are detected by their thermal reflect. Their wave lengths are longer than those of visible light and shorter than those of radio waves. (9) Ultraviolet Therapy, Outside the visible spectrum at its violet end; said of rays more refrangible than the extreme violet rays and opposed to infrared. (10) Ear irrigations, (11) X-rays and Fluoroscopy, (12) Endo or electrocardiogram. A tracing made by means of the electric needle of an electrocardiograph which shows the contractions of the heart muscle. (13) Special interpretations, (14) Laboratory examinations, (15) Physical examinations, (16) Basal Metabolism, the changes going on continually in living cells, by which energy is provided for vital processes and activities in the body, and new material is produced to repair the waste. (17) Hydro-Therapy Mineral baths. (18) Blood Count-Urine."

Moreover, appellants sent out literature to other chiropractors offering to do laboratory work and, among other things, they stated: "you no longer have to send your patient or children to other doctors to be treated for stomach worms or pin-worms. Read the enclosed bulletin on the one-week treatment and medication, you may legally give your patient for the above infestations."

It will be noticed that they advise other chiropractors to give "medications". They also furnished forms in connection with taking urine specimens in which they indicate that they could diagnose many diseases, including cancer, by examination of the urine. All this adds up to the fact that appellants did not confine their practice to that of chiropractic, but also engaged in the practice of medicine.

Ark. Stats. §72-407 gives the Chiropractic Board authority to revoke appellant's license "for prescribing any form of medical treatment without having first complied with the law governing the practice of medicine or any method which is not chiropractic." There is no showing that appellants have complied with the law governing the practice of medicine, and not only is their substantial evidence, but by a great weight of the evidence appellants prescribed treatments and methods of treatment which are not chiropractic.

(6) The Chiropractic Board's authority to revoke a license is not an arbitrary one; such authority must be exercised in a proper manner. Ark. Stats § 72-407 gives the Board authority to revoke a license on certain specified grounds, one of which is "prescribing any form of medical treatment." Here, when any and everything that may have been said in appellants absence is wholly disregarded, there remains overwhelming evidence that appellants engaged in the practice of medicine, and it is an aggravated case. The evidence shows that over a considerable period of time members of the Chiropractic

Board had attempted, without success, to get appellants to confine their practice to chiropractic. In this case, if the Board had failed to revoke the license on evidence which is properly in the record, there would have been an abuse of authority.

The judgment is affirmed.

DAVIS ET AL
v.
BEELER
Exhibit V
Attorney General, et al.
(*Supreme Court of Tennessee*. Nov. 29, 1947)
(*Rehearing Denied* Jan. 16, 1948)
(*Appeal Dismissed March* 27, 1948)
See 68 S.Ct. 745

1. Statutes - 215
In construing a statute to ascertain legislative intent, it is permissible to take note of conditions existing at time of such an enactment.

2. Physicians And Surgeons - 1
The Legislature has right to require a general practitioner's license for those who desire to practice a limited branch of the healing arts.

3. Physicians And Surgeons - 2
The statute repealing prior statute authorizing licensing of naturopath and prohibiting practice of naturopathy in state would be treated as one imposing additional qualifications upon persons already in practice of the profession. Pub. Acts 1943 c. 49,§ 4, as amended by Pub. Acts 1945, c. 43; Pub. Acts 1947, c. 2, §§ 1, 2.

4. Statutes - 225

The statute repealing prior statute authorizing licensing of naturopaths and prohibiting practice in naturopathy in state discloses an effort on part of Legislature to regulate one phase of the healing arts, and should be construed in pari materia with other statutes upon such subject. Pub. Acts 1947, c.2 §§ 1, 2.

5. Statutes - 225

Statutes forming a system or scheme should be construed so as to make that scheme consistent in all its parts and uniform in its operation.

6. Physicians And Surgeons - 2

The statute repealing prior statute authorizing licensing of naturopaths and prohibiting practice of naturopathy in state, when construed as not prohibiting use of such methods by one having a general practitioner's license or license to practice osteopathy, is a valid exercise of police power, and is not invalid as discriminatory against naturopaths and in favor of osteopaths and chiropractors. Pub. Acts 1947, c.2, §§ 1, 2.

On Petition to Rehear

7. Constitutional Law - 70 (3)

Supreme Court does not have function to disturb motives of legislative body in enacting legislation within its power.

8. Physicians And Surgeons 11 (1)

Physician's right to practice is a "property right" of which he cannot be arbitrarily deprived.

See Words and Phrases, Permanent Edition, for all other definitions of "Property Rights."

9. Physicians And Surgeons - 1

Physician's right to practice is a qualified one, held in subordination to duty of state under police power to protect public health.

10. Constitutional Law - 61

Police power cannot be stipulated or bartered away.

11. Constitutional Law - 62
Physicians and Surgeons - 1

Legislature may prescribe qualifications for those who practice medicine and may regulate drugless healers, which regulatory power may be properly committed to an administrative board or officer.

12. Constitutional Law - 199

Regulatory statutes may be made operative on those engaged in practice prior to their enactment, and may make qualifications more rigid from time to time.

13. Constitutional Law - 199

Legislature may prescribe qualifications as to character and learning which will require those in practice to give up their occupation, subject only to limitation that regulation be reasonable and bear some relation to service to be rendered by practitioner.

14. Constitutional Law - 82

A "bill of attainder" is a legislative act which inflicts punishment without a judicial trial.

See Words and Phrases, Permanent Edition, for all other definitions of "Bill of Attainder".

15. Constitutional Law - 82
Physicians And Surgeons - 2

The statute repealing prior statute authorizing licensing of naturopaths and prohibiting practice of naturopathy in state is not invalid as a ''bill of attainder'' Pub. Acts 1947, c.2, §§ 1, 2.

16. Constitutional Law - 197

An ''ex post facto law'' is one making an act, innocent when done, criminal and inflicting punishment, or aggravating crime, making it greater than it was when committed, or which changes punishment, inflicting greater punishment than was prescribed when committed, or which alters rules of evidence and receives less or different testimony than was required to convict at time of commission of offense.

See Words and Phrases, Permanent Edition, for all other definitions of ''Ex Post Facto Law.''

Error to Chancery Court, Davidson County; Thos. A. Shirver, Chancellor.

Suit by W. E. Davis and others against Roy H. Beeler, Attorney General, and others, to determine validity of statute dealing with practice of naturopathy in the state. To review adverse decree, the complainants bring error.

Reversed.

Goodpasture, Carpenter & Dale, of Nashville, for complainants.

Nat Tipton, Asst. Atty. Gen., for defendants.

PREWITT, Justice.

The purpose of the bill filed in this cause was to determine the validity of Chapter 2 of the Public Acts of 1947. This Act deals with the practice of naturopathy in this State. Section 1 of the Act repeals the Act authorizing the licensing of naturopaths, and Section 2 prohibits the practice of naturopathy in this State.

The chancellor upheld the validity of Section 1 of the Act, but struck down section 2 because it constituted an unwarranted abuse of the police power of the Legislature and held that naturopathy, being a lawful vocation, could not be prohibited but could only be regulated.

The effect of the chancellor's decree is to remove from the Code the provisions as to licensing of applicants to practice naturopathy, but to leave in effect the licenses granted from 1943 to 1947. It appears that there are some two hundred licensed naturopaths in the State at the present time.

(1) In construing a statute to ascertain the legislative intent, it is permissible to take note of the conditions existing at the time of such an enactment. It appears that at the session of the General Assembly previous to the one enacting this statute, a committee was appointed to investigate the unlawful practice of the healing arts, and that the committee made a report to the General Assembly enacting the statute. The report revealed that licenses to practice naturopathy had been issued to wholly unqualifed individuals; that they had been purchased; that they had been issued as a result of fraudulent co-operation; that a number of corporations had been chartered by naturopaths to issue certificates of compliance with the educational requirements of existing statutes; and that some of these chartered schools issued diplomas to persons who had attended the schools for a period of time not in excess of one week, but which diplomas certified that the holders thereof were qualified in a number of subjects dealing with the healing arts.

Appellants do not contend that the practices which go to constitute the practice of naturopathy are without the benefit in appropriate cases. They take the position further that nothing in the statute in question undertakes to outlaw them nor to prohibit their use by qualified persons.

Naturopathy as defined in Chapter 49 of the Acts of 1943, as amended, Williams' Code, §7025.4, as follows:

"By this Act Naturopathy is permitted to be practiced in the State of Tennessee under the provisions of this Act when a person is so qualified, and means, 'Nature cure or health by natural methods; and is defined as the prevention, diagnosis, and treatment of human injuries, ailments, and diseases by the use of such physical forces, as air, light, water, vibration, heat, electricity, hydrotherapy, psychotherapy, dietetics, or massage, and the administration of botanical and biological drugs, but shall not include the administration of narcotics, sulfa drugs and other toxic drugs, or powerful physical agents, such as X-ray and radium therapy, or surgery, the 'minor matters' mentioned in Section 12 (§ 7025.12) of this act to be construed as not including tonsillectomy, the opening of the thoracic or abdominal cavities or other major operations requiring an incision. Provided, that this bill or any language shall not apply to, or in any way affect Medical Doctors." Pub. Acts 1945 c.43.

No doubt, in the enactment of the Act now under consideration by us, the Legislature was seeking to cure the evils connected with the issuance of licenses to practice naturopathy, and in view of the fact that investigations disclosed that these licenses had been issued in a number of cases to persons totally unqualified was to take steps against the holders of such licenses, and not to outlaw the acts constituting such.

The Act contains no prohibition against the performance of these acts, but merely makes it unlawful for such persons to practice naturopathy.

As we conceive the legislature intent, as gathered from the fact of the statute and from conditions existing at the time, is that the prohibition leveled by it was directed at the persons engaged in the practice of naturopathy in this State, and that this legislative purpose was evidenced first, by a bar to all future licensing of such and second, by a prohibition against the use of the licenses theretofore issued. The legislative attempt, in enacting the statute under consideration, was to prevent the practice of naturopathy by ones having only limited qualifications and not possessing what might be termed a general practitioner's or osteopath's certificate, and it cannot be held that the Legislature intended to prohibit the performance of the acts.

(2-4) Physicians are licensed under Chapter 181 of the Public Acts of 1945, and osteopaths under Section 7003 et.seq. of Williams' Code. No prohibition exists against these generally licensed practitioners from performing the acts in question and when the three statutory schemes are read together and as a while, it appears that the Legislature does not deny to osteopaths or general practitioners the right to use methods employed by the complainants but simply sought to regulate the employment of these methods and to confine them to those having a general qualification. The effect of the statute governing the practice of medicine, the practice of osteopathy, and the present statute is that no person shall practice naturopathy unless he be licensed either as a general practitioner or as an osteopath. It cannot be disputed that the Legislature has the right to require a general practitioner's license for those who desire to practice a limited branch of the healing arts. The present statute may be treated as one imposing additional qualifications upon persons already in the practice of the profession. Hawker v. New York 170 U.S. 189, 18 S.Ct. 573, 42 L.Ed. 1002; Reetz v. Michigan, 188 U.S. 505, 23 S.Ct. 390, 47 L.Ed. 563. The present statute discloses an effort on the part of the Legislature to regulate one phase of the healing arts and should be construed in pari materia with other statutes upon this subject.

(5) In Howard and Herrin v. N.C. & St. L. Ry. Co., 153 Tenn. 649, 660, 284 S.W.894, 897, 46 A.L.R. 1530, the Court said:

"Statutes forming a system or scheme should be construed so as to make that scheme consistent in all its parts and uniform in its operation, Harris v. State, 96 Tenn. 496, 34 S.W.1017; (Stonega) Coke & Coal Co. v. (Southern) Steel Co. 123 Tenn. 428, 131 S.W. 988, 31 L.R.A., N.S. 278; Bird v. State, 131 Tenn. 518, 175 S.W.554, Ann. Cas. 1917A, 634. All acts in peri materia should be taken together as if one law. Merriman v. Lacefield, 51 Tenn. 209."

Nowhere in this statute or in any of the related statutes can there be found prohibition against the use of these methods by persons otherwise qualified and licensed to use them. By obtaining a general practitioner's license or license to practice osteopathy, persons may pursue the practice naturopathy without legal restraint. Stated in another way, this statute merely required that persons desiring to practice naturopathy shall obtain a general practitioner's license or one to practice osteopathy. Such a construction permits the science to be used by general practitioners and by osteopaths. The statute in question is aimed at the practitioners and not at the science. (The evident intent of the Legislature was to withdraw recognition of naturopathy as a separate branch of the healing arts but allow the use of its methods.) (Any person now licensed to practice naturopathy may continue the use of such methods by obtaining the additional knowledge required to qualify as a general practitioner or as an osteopath.)

In Commonwealth v. Zimmerman, 221 Mass. 184, 108 N.E. 893, 895, Ann. Cas. 1916A, 858, the Supreme Court of Massachusetts, in sustaining such requirement, gives its reason as follows:

"...The protection of the public from those who undertake to treat or manipulate the human body without the degree of education, training, and skill which the Legislature has prescribed as necessary to the general safety of the people is within the police power of the state. This general purpose may be effectuated by requiring even those who propose to confine their practice to a narrow specialty a much broader knowledge of the subject provided such qualification is regarded by the Legislature as necessary for the practice of any branch of medicine. The statute does not impair in any constitutional sense the liberty of the defendant. The protection of the public health is an object of such vital importance to the welfare of the state that any rational means to that end must be upheld."

In State v. Smith, 233 No. 242, 135 S.W. 465, 472, the same insistence was made and rejected by the Supreme Court of Missouri in the following language:

"...The Legislature thought, perhaps, that this act was necessary to protect credulous sick people from injury at the hands of charlatans and quacks, with their specious promises of a sure cure without drugs; or it may have been thought necessary to forbid harmless practices in order to insure protection against those that are dangerous and harmful. Sick people sometimes grow desperate in their search for a cure, or their judgment becomes weakened, so that they fall an easy prey to the ingenious and varied devices of the pretended healer."

Dr. Herzog in his work on Medical Jurisprudence very clearly calls attention to the dangers flowing from the limited knowledge of the limited practitioner as follows:

"While electro-therapy, mechano-therapy, hydrotherapy, suggestive therapeutics, and certain other forms of treatment for which licenses are issued to limited practitioners are valuable in many pathological conditions, the limited practitioner is likely to do a great deal of harm, not only because he is not thoroughly educated as a physician but as he is only licensed to use certain system of treatment, he is apt to use it in cases to which it is not adapted."

Obviously, a much more accurate diagnosis may be expected from a general practitioner who has studied medicine and disease in all its phases than from a limited one with only limited preparation therefore, and an accurate diagnosis of an ailment lies at the very foundation of successful methods of treatment.

The choice of the remedy to be applied to the evil

rests with the Legislature and not with the courts, these being co-ordinate branches of government.

But it is insisted that what has been indicated herein will render the statute discriminatory against naturopaths and in favor of osteopaths and chiproactors.

In Louisiana State Board of Medical Examiners v. Fife, 162 La. 681, 111 So. 58, 61,54 A.L.R. 594, affirmed by U.S. Supreme Court in 274 U.S. 720, 47 S.Ct. 590, 71 L.Ed. 1324, the Supreme Court of Louisiana said:

"...If the Legislature were called upon to recognize every school of medicine, and to deal with it as such, requiring nothing but what the system practiced by each school demands, there might be some force to defendant's contention, but, as we have held, the Legislature is not called upon to do so, but has a reasonable discretion as to whether a particular school should be recognized and special provision made for it. Since the Legislature has such discretion, defendants cannot complain, on the ground of being unjustly discriminated against, because the Legislature has not deemed proper to recognize their school of medicine, and make special provision for those desiring to practice that system, by prescribing a course of study in accord with the theories which it holds for restoring health. See Allopathic State Board of Medical Examiners v. Fowler, supra. (50 La.Ann. 1358, 24 So. 809); Johnson v. State, Tex: Civ. App. 267 S.W. 1057; Singh v. State, 66 Tex. Cr.R 156, 146 S.W.891; State, Tex. Civ. App. , 267 S.W. 1057; Singh "5".

Section 7004 of Williams' Code requires that osteopaths shall successfully pass an examination upon virtually all subjects within the purview of medical science. Furthermore, the qualifications for osteopaths are sub-

stantially the same as those required by general practitioners. No doubt the Legislature thought that the profi-
ciency in the healing arts was sufficient to authorize them
to practice generally.

As to chiropractors, they are required to show evidence of having studied certain medical subjects for an
extended period too, and the statute authorizing them to
practice their treatment is restricted to manual manipulation of the spine and adjacent tissues. Naturopaths were
not so restricted in their treatment of diseases but might
treat them generally with the exception of surgery and
the administration of toxic and powerful drugs. It is not
difficult to see, considering the areas in which they
oeprate, why the Legislature would demand higher educational requirements for naturopaths than are required
for chiroprators.

After all, why should not persons who hold themselves out to be doctors, who not only rub and massage
patients but prescribe medicine for them, even though
narcotics and sulfa drugs are prohibiited, be required to
have the training of a medical doctor? Evidently, the Legislature thought there was too much border-lining in the
practice of naturopathy and determined to stamp out the
evil that was not in the science but in the practicing of it,
to the definite injury of credulous sufferers.

In Zahn v. Board of Public Works, 274 U.S. 325, 328,
47 S.Ct. 594, 595, 71 L.Ed.1074, 1076, the Supreme
Court of the United States said:

"...The most that can be said is that whether that
determination was an unreasonable, arbitrary, or une-
qual exercise of power is fairly debatable. In such circumstances, the settled rule of this court is that it will not

substitute its judgment for that of the legislative body charged with the primary duty and responsibility of determining the question. Euclid v. Ambler Realty Co., supra (272, U.S. 365), pages 388, 395, (396), 47 S.Ct. 114 (71 L.Ed. 303, 54A.L.R. 1016); Radice v. New York, 264 U.S. 292, 294, 44 S.Ct. 325, 68 L.Ed.690 (694); Hadacheck v. Sebastian 239 U.S. 394, 408, 412-414, 36 S.Ct. 143, 60 L.Ed.348 (355-358). Ann. Cas. 1917B, 927; Thomas Cusack Co. v. Chicago, 242 U.S. 526, 530, 531, 37 S.Ct. 190, 61 L.Ed. 472, (475, 476), L.R.A. 1918A, 136, Ann. Cas. 1917C, 594; Rast v. Van Deman & L. Co. 240 U.S. 342, 357, 36 S.Ct., 370, 60 L.Ed., 679 (687), L.R.A. 1917A, 421, Ann. Cas. 1917B, 455; Price v. Illinois, 238 U.S. 466, 452, 35 S.Ct. 892, 59 L.Ed. 1400 (1405)."

(6) It results that we are of opinion that the enactment in question prohibiting naturopathy in this State is a valid exercise of the police power of the Legislature and no unwarranted discrimination appears in the Act.

The decree of the Chancellor is accordingly reversed as in our opinion, Section 2 of the Act is a valid enactment.

NEIL, C.J. and GAILOR and TOMLINSON, JJ., concur

BURNETT, J. not participating.

On Petition to Rehear

PREWITT, Justice

A petition to rehear has been filed herein, but a number of the matters complained of were fully considered by the Court in our former opinion.

(7) We held the legislation in question to be within the police power of the Legislature, and this being true, it becomes immaterial what portion of the regulated pro-

fession requires safeguards, as it is not a function of Court to disturb the motives of a legislative body in enacting legislation within its power.

(8-13) The law applicable to the power of the Legislature in regulating branches of the healing arts is well expressed in the case of Butcher v. Maybury, D.C., 8 F.2d 155, 158, 159, as follows:

The right of a physician to practice his profession is a property right, of which he cannot be arbitrarily deprived. Dent v. West Virginia, 129 U.S. 114, 123, 124, 9 S.Ct. 231, 32 L.Ed. 623; Douglas v. Noble, 261 U.S. 165, 43 S.Ct. 303, 67 L.Ed. 590; Bogni v. Perotti, 224 Mass. 152, 112 N.E. 853, 855, L.R.A. 1916F, 831; Lawrence v. Board of Registration, 239 Mass. 424, 132 N.E. 174, 176; State v. Medical Board, 32 Minn. 324, 20 N.W. 238, 50 Am.Rep. 575, 576.

"The right is a qualified one, and is held in subordination to the duty of the state under the police power to protect the public health. Hawker v. New York 170 U.S. 189, 18 S.Ct. 573, 42 L.Ed. 1002, Lawrence v. Board of Registration, 239 Mass. 424, 132 N.E. 174, 176. The police power cannot be stipulated or bartered away. Gray v. Connecticut 159 U.S. 74, 15 S.Ct. 985, 40 L.Ed. 80. In State v. Hovorka, 100 Minn. 249, 252, 110 N.W. 870, 871, 8 L.R.A., N.S., (1272), 1273, 1275. 10 Ann. Cas. 398, it is said:

"No person can acquire a vested right to continue, when once licensed, in a business, trade, or occupation which is subject to legislative control and regulation under the police power. The rights and liberty of the citizen are all held in subordination to that governmental prerogative, and to such reasonable regulations and restrictions as the Legislature may from time to time prescribe. * * * Regulations so prescribed and conformed to by the citizen may be subsequently changed or modified by the Legislature, whenever public interest require it, without subjecting its action to the charge of interfering with contract or vested rights. This is elementary.

"In a note found on page 1273 of 8 L.R.A., N.S., the author says:

"The granting of a license in such cases is merely the means taken by the state, in the exercise of its police power, to regulate and restrict the engaging in certain professions and occupations for the public good, and confers no rights whatever, in the way of a contract with the state, upon the licensee. He takes the same subject to the right of the state, at any time that the public good demands, to make further restrictions and regulations thereto; and, if such restrictons and regulations are reasonable, they will be upheld, even though they may actually prohibit some people from further engaging in such occupations or professions under a license previously granted."

"The authorities held without dissent that it is competent for the Legislature to prescribe qualifications for those who are to practice medicine and thus to assure that they shall possess the requisite character and learning. Dent v. West Virginia, 129 U.S. 114, 122, 9 S.Ct. 231, 32 L.Ed. 623; Hawker v. New York 170 U.S. 189, 18 S.Ct. 573; 42 L.Ed, 1002; State v. State Medical Board, 32 Minn., 324, 20 N.W. 238, 50 Am. Rep. 575, 577. The regulation of drugless healers is a proper exercise of the police power. Crane v. Johnson, 242 U.S. 339, 37 S.Ct. 176, 61 L.Ed. 348, Ann. Cas. 1917B, 796. The regulatory power of the state may be properly committed to an administrative board or officer. Douglas v. Noble, 261 U.S. 165, 170, 43 S.Ct. 303, 67 L.Ed. 590; State v. State Medical Board, 32 Minn. 324, 20 N.W. 238, 50 Am. Rep.575,577.

"These regulatory statutes may be made operative on those engaged in practice prior to the enactment of the statutes. Dent v. West Virginia, 129 U.S. 114, 122, 9 S.Ct. 231, 32, L.Ed. 623; Collins v. Texas, 223 U.S. 288, 295, 32S.Ct., 286, 56 L.Ed. 439; Lawrence v. Board of Registration, 239 Mass. 424, 132 N.E., 174, 176. The state may change the qualifications from time to time, making them more rigid. Dent v. West Virginia, 129 U.S. 114, 122, 9 S.Ct. 231, 32 L.Ed. 623; Gray v. Connecticut, 159 U.S. 74, 15 S.Ct., 985, 40 L.Ed. 80; State v. Hovorka, 100 Minn. 249, 110 N.W. 870, 8 L.R.A., N.S. (1272), 1273, 1275, 10 Ann. Cas. 398.

"The Legislature may prescribe qualifications both as to character and learning, which will require those in practice to give up their occupation. Dent v. West Virginia, 129 U.S. 114, 122, 9 S.Ct. 231, 32 L.Ed. 123; Hawker v. New York, 170 U.S. 189, 8 S.Ct. 573, 42 L.Ed. 1002. Legislation prescribing qualifications which a practitioner cannot meet because of conditions antedating the enactment of the legislation is valid. Such legislation does not constitute punishment, it is legitimate regulation. Hawker v. New York, 170 U.S. 189, 18 S.Ct.573, 42 L.Ed. 1002, Meffert v. State Board of Medical Registration, 66 Kan. 710, 72P, 247, 1 L.R.A. N.S., 811."

The authorities mentioned in the case quoted above disclose that it lies within the police power to require educational qualifications of those already engaged in the practice of any profession.

(14-16)The insistence that the Act is in the nature of a bill of attainder is answered by Butcher v. Maybury, supra, where the same insistence was made. The reply to this insistence in that case is as follows at pages 159, 160 of 8 F.2d:

"'A bill of attainder is a legislative act which inflicts punishment without a judicial trial.' Cummings v. Missouri, 4 Wall. 277, 323, 18 L.Ed. 356. The statute in question inflicts no punishment. Meffert v. State Board of Medical Registration, 66 Kan. 710, 72 P. 247, 251, 1 L.R.A., N.S. 811; Hawker v. New York, 170 U.S. 189, 18 S.Ct., 573, 42 L.Ed. 1002. If plaintiffs lose the right to continue the practice of their profession, it will not be as a punishment for some offense committed by them, but because their qualifications do not measure up to the legislative requirements.

"In Calder v. Bull, Pa. 3 Dall, 386, 390, 1 L.Ed. 648, the court classifies ex post facto laws as follows:

"'(1) Every law that makes an action done before the passing of the law, and which was innocent when done, criminal, and punishes such action.

"' (2) Every law that aggravates a crime, or makes it greater than it was when committed.

"'(3) Every law that changes the punishment, and inflicts a greater punishment than the law annexed to the crime, when committed.

"'(4) Every law that alters the legal rules of evidence and receives less, or different, testimony, than the law required at the time of the commission of the offense, in order to convict the offender.'

"This definition has been repeatedly approved in form or substance. Hopt v. Utah, 110 U.S. 574, 589 4 S.Ct. 202, 28 L.Ed. 262; Mallett v. North Carolina, 181 U.S. 589, 593, 21S.Ct.730, 45 L.Ed.1015; Kentucky Union Co. v. Kentucky, 219 U.S. 140, 31 S.Ct. 171, 55 L.Ed. 137. It is manifest that the statute in question does not fall within the above classification. It has been expressly held that a statute which makes provisions for the cancellation of licenses of those engaged in the practice of medicine is not obnoxious to the ex post facto provision of the Federal Constitution. Reetz v. Michigan, 188 U.S. 505, 510, 23 S.Ct. 390, 47 L.Ed., 563."

After careful consideraton of the petition to rehear, we are convinced that the Legislature was well within its powers in enacting the statute prohibiting the practice of naturopathy in this State. The methods employed by naturopaths may still be used by those formerly practicing naturoapthy if they obtain the qualifications now possessed by medical doctors and osteopaths.

It results that the petition to rehear is denied.

All concur.

Exhibit VI
DR. JOSEPH W. HOWE,
DR. MICHAEL A. GIAMMARINO, AND
PENNSYLVANIA LICENSED CHIROPRACTORS,
ASSOCIATION, APPELLANTS
v.
THEODORE B. SMITH, JR., HARRY H. BRAINERD,
AND H. EARL PITZER.
(*Superior Court of Pennsylvania, April 14, 1964.*)

Proceeding by chiropractors and chiropractors' association to enjoin Secretary of Revenue and his subordinates from refusing to accept certificates from chiropractors concerning physical fitness of motor vehicle oeprators. The Court of Common Pleas of Dauphin County, as of Equity No. 2559, No 544, Commonwealth Docket 1962, Walter R. Sohn, President Judge, entered order dismissing the complaint, and the plaintiffs appealed. The Superior Court, No. 60 March Term, 1964, Woodside, J. held that Secretary of Revenue who accepted physical examinations of motor vehicle operators by physicians but not examinations by chiropractors was exercising discretion given him by Legislature and was not unconstitutionally discriminating between the two professions.

Order affirmed.

1. Physicians And Surgeons - 6 (1)
Limited license issued under Medical Practice Act provision permitting licensing of chiropractors does not authorize licensee to practice medicine or healing arts generally. 63 P.S.§§ 401, 408.

2. Constitutional Law - 238 (1)

Secretary of Revenue who accepted physical examinations of motor vehicle operators by physicians but not examinations by chiropractors was exercising discretion given him by Legislature and was not unconstitutionally discriminating between the two professions, in view of real distinction between physicians and chiropractors as recognized by Legislature. 46 P.S. §601; 63 P.S. §§ 401, 408, 601, 602(b), 605; 75 P.S. §608(g); P.S. Const. art. 1,§ 1; U.S.C.A. Const. Amend. 14.

3. Constitutional Law - 208 (1)

Classifications for purposes of legislating is permissible. P.S Const. art. 1,§ 1. U.S.C.A. Const. Amend. 14.

4. Statutes - 77 (1)

Act which applies to all members of class is general, not special. P.S. Const. art. 3,§ 7.

5. Constitutional Law - 208 (6)
Physicians and Surgeons - 2

Legislative classification distinguishing between physicians and chiropractors is constitutional in view of substantial distinction between treatment offered and significant difference in education and training required. P.S.Const. art. 1,§ 1; U.S.C.A.Const. Amend. 14.

Jacob S. Richman, Philadelphia, for appellants.

W. E. Shissler, Nauman, Smith, Shissler & Hall, Harrisburg, for Dr. J. M. Clarke, Dr. D. A. Gipson, Dr. G. Harry Lewis and Dr. W. Fogle, amici curiae.

William M. Gross, Joseph L. Cohen, Asst. Atts. Gen., Walter E. Alessandroni, Att. Gen. Harrisburg for appellee.

Before RHODES, P. J., and ERVIN, WRIGHT, WOOD-SIDE, WATKINS, MONTGOMERY and FLOOD, JJ.

WOODSIDE, Judge

This is an appeal from the dismissal of an amended complaint in equity to enjoin the Secretary of Revenue and his administrative subordinates from refusing to accept certificates from chiropractors concerning the physical fitness of certain motor vehicle operators.

Two duly licensed chiropractors and the Pennsylvania Licensed Chiropractors' Association filed a complaint in equity in the Dauphin County Court of Common Pleas, sitting as the Commonwealth Court. The plaintiffs alleged that the Secretary of Revenue and the other defendants have unlawfully discriminated against licensed chiropractors by refusing to accept their certificates of the physical fitness of their patients.

The Attorney General filed preliminary objections in the nature of a demurrer. The court below accepted the Attorney General's contention that the amended complaint did not set forth a cause of action and dismissed it. The plaintiffs appealed, contending that we should remand the case for disposition after hearing, or, at least, permit them to further amend the complaint in order to more clearly, fully and sharply plead the scope of practice of the plaintiffs as authorized by statute and the professional boards' regulations.

Accepting as true all of the facts (but not the conclusions of law and suggested interpretations of statutes) set forth in the amended complaint, we agree with the court below that it does not set forth a cause of action, and that all the facts necessary to a determination of the issue are before us. As we view it, nothing could be gained by the plaintiffs were they to be given a hearing or allowed to further amend their complaint.

The complaint sets forth that in 1960 the secretary instituted a program requiring applicants for motor vehicle learner's permits and operator's licenses and certain licensed operators to submit to an examination by a licensed physician as a condition to obtaining or retaining their operating privileges.[1]

1. According to the appellants' brief, "the examination encompassed ten conditions to be checked: four, by the State Police such as (1)loss of use of both hands; (2) neurological disorders affecting musuclar control and coordination to a noticeable degree; (3) 20/70 vision or less; (4) dyspnea—obvious shortness of breath on slight exertion; and six, by a licensed physician—(1) hypertension; (2) neuropsychiatric disorders causing substantial disturbances; (3) conditions causing lapses of consciousness; (4) uncontrolled diabetes; (5)chronic alcoholism, (6) drug addiction."

In requiring the examination, the secretary acted pursuant to the authority contained in § 608(g) of The Vehicle Code of April 29, 1959, P.L. 58, 75 P.S. § 608(g), which provides: "The secretary may, in his discretion, require the special examination by such agencies as the secretary may direct, of any applicant for learner's permit or operator's license, or of any operator, to determine incompetency, physical or mental disability or disease, or any other condition which might prevent such applicant from exercising reasonable and ordinary control over a motor vehicle or tractor."

The plaintiffs do not question the validity of the secretary's authority to require physical and mental examinations of licensees or applicants for licenses, but they contend that by limiting the examinations to physicians and refusing to accept the certificates of chiroporactors, the secretary is discriminating against them in violation of the Equal Protection Clauses of the 14th Amendment of the United States Constitution, and Article 1, Section 1 of the Pennsylvania Constitution, P.S.

The Commonwealth Court, in an opinion by President Judge Walter R. Sohn, decided that only licensed physicians had the statutory authority to diagnose diseases, and that determining mental disabilities and diagnosing diseases are in the area that is prohibited to the practice of chiropractic. Of course, if the chiropractors may not diagnose, the secretary was not only authorized but required to reject all certificates of examination made by them.

(1) Chiropractors were first licensed to practice their profession in Pennsylvania under the Medical Practice Act of June 3, 1911, P. L. 639, as amended, 63 P.S. §§. 401, 408. This is the act providing for the licensing of medical practitioners, as well as others engaged in the healing arts. Plaintiff Giammarino was admitted to practice under this act. It contains no definition of chiropractor or chiropractic, but it provides not only for the issuance of medical licenses but also for the issuance of certificates "Limited to the practice of his or her pursuit" for which the person was specifically licensed. Limited licenses issued under this act do not authorize the licensee to practice medicine or the healing arts generally. Commonwealth v. Allison, 155 Pa. Super. 290, 38 A.2d 535 (1944).

The Chiropractic Registration Act of August 10, 1951, P.L. 1182, 63 P.S. § 601 et seq, dealt with chiropractic and provided for the licensing of chiropractors. This act is § 2(b), 63 P.S. § (602b) defines Chiropractic as "a system of locating misaligned or displaced vertebrae of the human spine, the examination preparatory to and the adjustment by hand of such misaligned or displaced vertebrae, and other articulations, together with the use of scientific instruments of analysis, as taught in the approved schools and colleges of chiropractic, without the use of either drugs or surgery. The term 'chiropractic' shall not include the practice of obstetrics or reduction of fractures or major dislocations." Plaintiff Howe is licensed under this act.

Section 13 of the Chiropractic Registration Act, 63 P.S. § 613, provides that practitioners, such as plaintiff Giammarino, "licensed or legally authorized to practice chiropractic" under the Act of 1911 shall continue to possess the same rights and privileges with respect o the practice of chiropractic without being required to be licensed anew under the provisions of the Act of 1951.

A comparison of the provisions of the Medical Practice Act of 1911, supra, relating to the practice of medicine and surgery with the provisions of the Chiropractic Registration Act of 1951, supra, shows the different educational requirements, different rights and different duties established for chiropractors and for those licensed to practice medicine and surgery. The validity of the prohibition against chiropractors practicing medicine is not and cannot be denied.

The plaintiffs admit that their right to treat diseases is limited, but they contend that the Chiropractic Registration Act authorizes them to diagnose diseases without limit, and hence the examination required to certify the fitness of an applicant for an operator's license is within their statutory powers. They argue that the legislature indicated its intent to authorize them to diagnose diseases generally by including in the statutory definition of chiropractic "locating misalignment" and "the examination preparatory to" adjustment, "together with the use of scientific instruments of analysis." If it was the intent of the legislature to authorize the chiropractor to diagnose generally it certainly did not spell it out as clearly as it could have and should have. In fact the very use of the word "preparatory" indicates the examination was to be related to the limited practice of "adjustment". The legislature used the expression "diagnose diseases" in the Medical Practice Act, *supra*, in a provision which says, "It shall not be lawful for any person...to diagnose diseases...excepting those hereinafter exempted, unless...(he) has received a certificate of licensure" under the Act 63 P.S. § 401a. If the chiropractors believe that they are trained and qualified to diagnose diseases without restriction, they should ask the legislature to grant them that right rather than seek to have the courts confer it upon them by a strained construction of the statutes.

Of course, chiropractors may and must diagnose before they treat. However, in their argument here they have failed to recognize the obvious distinction between the authority to diagnose generally and the authority to diagnose for the limited purpose of determining whether the particular treatment which they may legally render to a patient is proper treatment for the disease from which the patient is suffering.

The apellants point to the educational requirements of the chiropractors as the basis for their ability to diagnose diseases generally. We have no doubt that many chiropractors have extensive knowledge and training. There, too, are many admitted to practice whose required formal education was far less than that required of medical practitioners, and even present applicants for a chiropractic license. This is especially true of those admitted under § 5 of the Chiropractic Registration Act, 63 P.S. § 605, a "grandfather clause."[2] Furthermore, there are techniques of diagnosis which a physician may use that are denied by statute to a chiropractor, for example, the use of diagnostic drugs.

By the amendment of June 14, 1957, P.L. 323, to cause 87 of §101 of the Statutory Construction Act of May 28, 1937, P.L. 1019, 46 P.S. § 601, the legislature redefined physician to mean, "an individual licensed under the laws of this Commonwealth to engage in the practice of medicine and surgery in all of its branches within the scope of the act, approved June 3, 1911, P.L. 639) and its amendments, or in the practice of osteopathy or osteopathic surgery within the scope of the act, approved (March 19, 1909, P.L. 46) and its amendments."

2. For definition of "grandfather clause" see In re Berman, 245 N.C. 612, 97 S.E.2d 232 (1957).

Naturally the chiropractors would like to be equated with the medical profession, but neither their recognized field of practice nor the statutes relating to these professions makes such an equation realistic. Chiropractors are engaged in a limited field of the healing arts which requires less education and training of them than is required of those practicing medicine and surgery. They are classified separately by the legislature from physicians in numerous ways.

(2) The Secretary of Revenue in accepting only examinations certified by physicians was recognizing a real distinction between physicians and chiropractors which has been recognized by the legislature. He was exercising the discretion given him by the legislature to have the examination made "by such agencies[3] as the secretary may direct."

(3-5) A classification of this nature made by the legislature or a governmental official does not violate the 14th Amendment to the Constitution of the United States nor Article 1, Section 1, nor Article 3, Section 7 of the Pennsylvania Constitution, as contended by the appellants. Classification for the purpose of legislating has been recognized as permissible under the Constitution of 1874 since Wheeler v. City of Philadelphia, 77 Pa. 338 (1875). An act which applies to all the members of the class is general and not special, and thus does not violate Article 3, Section 7 of the Pennsylvania Constitution. Commonwealth v. Hanley, 15 Pa. Super, 271, 280 (1900). It is only when the classification is not founded on real and substantial distinctions that it becomes unconstitutional. Young v. Department of Public Instruction, 105 PA super, 153, 159, 160 A. 151 (1932). There is a real and substantial distinction between the treatment offered by a chiropractor and that offered by a physician as defined in the Statutory Construction Act, supra. There is also a significant difference in the education and training required. The classification made by the legislature is constitutional. Commonwealth v. Allison, supra, 155 Pa. Super.

290, 38 A.2d, 535 (1944); Terenzio v. Devlin, 361 Pa. 602, 65 A.2d 374 (1949).

3. The plaintiffs contend that physicians are not an "agency," but they have no standing to raise that question, for if the secretary is limited to certificates from "agencies" as the plaintiffs wish us to construe the word, they themselves would not be an "agency" and hence unable to obtain the relief they seek.

The Secretary of Revenue in following the distinction between physicians and chiropractors recognized by the legislature was acting within the discretion given him by the legislature, and was not unconstitutionally discriminating between these professions,

Order affirmed

Exhibit VII
BETTY N. CORRELL, APPELLANT,
v.
J. M. GOODFELLOW, APPELLEE.

CHARLES CORRELL, APPELLANT,
v.
J. M. GOODFELLOW, APPELLEE,
No. 51104.
(*Supreme Court of Iowa. Jan. 14, 1964.*)

Malpractice actions against chiropractor. From judgment of the Pottawattamie District Court, Bennett Cullison, J. for the chiropractor on a directed verdict, the husband and wife appealed. The Supreme Court, Garfield, C. J., held that evidence including evidence that the diabetic wife's sprained ankle could have been successfully treated with an ultra-sonic machine but that injury did in fact result to her from the use of such machine made a case for the jury.

Reversed and remanded.

1. Physicians And Surgeons - 6 (1)

Use of such device as ultra-sonic machine on patients does not come within limited definition of chiropractic but constitutes part of practice of medicine and surgery. I.C.A. §§ 151.1 et seq., 151.1.

2. Courts - 107

Supreme Court's denial of plaintiff's appeal from ruling which denied permission to amend her petition was not approval of ruling but merely refusal to review it in advance of final judgment. 58 I.C.A. Rules of Civil Procedure, rules 118, 332(a).

3. Courts - 99 (2)

Where ruling denying first amendment was perhaps on ground it was untimely, and objection of untimeliness was not available as against second amendment, disallowance of first amendment was not law of case. 58 I.C.A. Rules of Civil Procedure, rule 118.

4. Pleading - 236 (2)

Trial court has a good deal of discretion in whether to allow amendment to pleading after responsive pleading has been filed. 58 I.C.A. Rules of Civil Procedure, rule 88.

5. Appeal And Error - 918 (1), 1201 (3)

Where law action is reversed and remanded on another ground than disallowance of amendment, trial court will have same discretion to permit amendment as if case had not been tried, and presumption is that after remand such discretion will not be abused. 58 I.C.A. Rules of Civil Procedure, rule 88.

6. Physicians And Surgeons - 14 (2)

Generally, one sued for malpractice is entitled to have his treatment tested by rules and principles of school of medicine to which he belongs and if he treats patient with ordinary skill and care of those of his school, he is not answerable for poor results, I.C.A. 151.1 et seq., 151.1.

7. Physicians And Surgeons - 14 (2)

In going outside practice of chiropractic and entering field of medicine by administering ultra-sonic treatments, chiropractor was held to care and skill usually exercised by medical doctors. I.C.A. §§ 151.1 et seq., 151.1.

8. Physicians And Surgeons - 15 (18)

Mere violation of statute relating to practice of chiropractor was not actionable negligence without proof that chiropractor failed to exercise proper care in treating plaintiff's foot and that such failure caused her injury. I.C.A. §§ 151.1 et seq., 151.1.

9. Trial - 178

In considering propriety of directed verdict for defendant, court would give evidence for plaintiff the most favorable construction it would reasonably bear.

10. Negligence - 136 (14, 25)

Generally, questions of negligence and proximate cause are for jury; they may be decided as matters of law only in exceptional cases. 58 I.C.A. Rules of Civil Procedure, rule 344(f), pars. 2, 10.

11. Physicians And Surgeons - 18 (8)

Testimony that if proper care were used a sprained ankle of diabetic could be successfully treated with ultrasonic machine, together with fact that injury resulted from treatment with such machine was some evidence that proper care and skill were not used. I.C.A. §§ 151.1 et seq., 151.1.

12. Trial - 98

Where objection to question was not made until after answer was in and no reason was given for delay, ruling sustaining objection did not have effect of striking testimony and the testimony remained in record to be considered.

13. Witnesses - 270 (2)

On trial of complaint that chiropractor failed to use such care in use of ultra-sonic machine as person skilled in such use was required to exercise, question, on cross-examination, whether use of doctor's prescription was generally accepted use of ultra-sonic machine in doctor's profession in the community was not objectionable under issue raised. I.C.A. §§ 151.1 et seq., 151.1.

14. Physicians And Surgeons - 18 (9)

In malpractice action against chiropractor, evidence including evidence that diabetic could have been successfully treated with ultra-sonic machine and that injury did in fact result from use of machine presented jury question of negligence. 58 I.C.A.§§ 151.1 et seq., 151.1.

15. Physicians And Surgeons - 18 (9)

Where there was ample evidence of chiropractor's negligence, issue of proximate cause was for jury. I.C.A.§§ 151.1 et seq., 151.1.

16. Negligence - 136 (25)

Issue of proximate cause is ordinarily for jury if there is substantial evidence of negligence.

Porter, Heithoff & Pratt, Council Bluffs, for appellants.

Smith, Peterson, Beckman & Willson, Council Bluffs, for appellee.

GARFIELD, *Chief Justice.*

Betty N. Correll, whom we call plaintiff, sued J. M. Goodfellow, a chiropractor in Council Bluffs, at law for alleged malpractice in burning her foot while treating it with an ultra-sonic machine. Betty's husband also sued defendant for alleged loss of consortium resulting from the injury. The cases were consolidated for trial. At the close of the evidence the trial court sustained generally defendant's motion for direct verdict which asserted, in effect, the evidence was insufficient to show plaintiff's injury was caused by any failure of defendant to exercise the requisite skill in applying the treatment. The appeal is from judgement on the directed verdict.

Plaintiff, 70 at the time of trial in May 1862, went to defendant September 26, 1960, for a sore back. She had been diabetic since 1948 and told defendant of her ailment. Defendant took x-rays of plaintiff's back, pronounced it in bad condition and assured her he treated diabetics. She purchased 12 treatments in order to save $6 from single treatment prices. Defendant treated plaintiff's back on September 26, 28 and 30.

Saturday, October 1, plaintiff turned her ankle and limped when she went to defendant for the treatment of her back on Monday, October 3. Defendant asked why she was limping, she replied she turned her ankle. Defendant said he had a machine which would take care of that. When he got out the ultra-sonic machine she said, "I'm diabetic, you wouldn't dare use that on my foot." Defendant assured her, "that won't bother you at all. You don't have that much diabetes." He proceeded to use the machine on her foot and repeated the treatment October 5th and 7th.

An ultra-sonic machine produces radiations which penetrate the tissue to cause internal vibrations which in turn causes heat to be generated deep inside the tissue. In fewer words, it is an electrical machine which produces heat by friction inside the tissue.

When defendant "plugged in" the machine plaintiff told him she didn't know chiropractors used those machines. He said, "I'm trying it out. I don't know anything yet about it, whether I want it or not. If it works I'm going to buy it. I won't buy it unless I know it works."

The second time defendant used the machine on plaintiff's foot it made the foot "so hot inside" and she so informed him. She went home "in such pain." Before plaintiff returned to defendant on October 7 her foot was blistered. She showed the blister to him and told him he caused it. So far as shown he made no denial. He treated the ankle the same on the 7th as on the two previous times. When plaintiff returned on October 10 she told defendant he could not "use that thing any more. Look what you did to my foot." There was a blister on the heel and across the bottom of the foot. Only the three ultra-sonic treatments were administered.

There is ample evidence plaintiff's foot was blistered and ulcerated from a burn or burns caused by defendant's use of the ultra-sonic machine. The injury was treated by a chiropodist-podiatrist in Omaha from October 15 to November 21 when he told plaintiff she must see her physician immediately. Plaintiff's physician took over treatment of the injury November 21. He sent her to a hospital January 8, 1961, where she was a patient until March 5. February 26 and March 1 the physician removed the back part of the injured heel. He testifed plaintiff has about 25 per cent permanent partial disability of the foot and perhaps 15 per cent permanent total disability of the foot and ankle.

We will refer later to evidence we think made the issues of defendant's alleged negligence, and that it was the proximate cause of plaintiff's injury, for the jury.

I. Plaintiff's petition (as well as the husband's) alleges defendant was negligent in administering the ultra-sonic machine and was not exercising that degree of skill usually exercised by chiropractors in Council Bluffs, defendant was incompetent to use the machine because of his own admission he was merely trying it out, and knew or should have known it should not have been applied to a diabetic.

Three months and 20 days after the petition was filed plaintiff filed an amendment thereto, adding to paragraph 3 thereof, just summarized, the allegation that defendant used the ultra-sonic machine in violation of chapter 151, Code, 1958, I.C.A. particularly section 151.1. Defendant resisted the amendment on four grounds: It was not timely; regulation of chiropractors is exclusively for the state; an individual cannot raise such a question; the amendment has no bearing on the standard of care required of defendant.

(1) Code chapter 151, I.C.A. regulates and limits the practice of chiropractic. So far as material here, section

151.1 defines persons engaged in such practice as "Persons who treat human ailments by the adjustment by hand of the articulations of the spine or by other incidental adjustments." This definition does not greatly differ from the well-known and generally accepted definition of chiropractic. State v. Boston, 226, Iowa 429, 436, 278 N.W. 291, 284 N.W. 143.

The use of such a device as an ultra-sonic machine on patients does not come within the limited definition of chiropractic but constitutes part of the practice of medicine and surgery. State v. Boston, supra; Joyner v. State, 181 Miss. 245, 179 So. 573, 115 A.L.R. 954, and Anno. 957-958; Treptau v. Behrens Spa, 247 Wis. 438, 20 N.W. 2d 108, 113; Anno, 86 A.L.R. 623, 630 ("A chiropractor cannot give electrical treatments without exceeding his authority." citations).

(2) The trial court, Judge Everest, denied plaintiff permission to so amend her petition. There was no separate ruling on each of the grounds of defendant's resistance as required by rule 118, Rules of Civil Procedure, 58 I.C.A. Nor does the record show the basis of the ruling.

Plaintiff applied to us under rule 332(a) R.C.P., to grant an appeal from the ruling. We denied the application. Such denial was not an approval of the ruling but merely a refusal, upon considerations we deemed sufficient, to review it in advance of final judgment. Deere Mfg. Co. v. Zeiner, 247 Iowa 1364, 1379, 78 N.W.2d 527, 79 N.W.2d 403, 404. See also Rubendall v. Brogan Constr. Co. 253 Iowa 652, 657, 113 N.W. 2d 265, 268.

Six months and ten days after the petition was filed plaintiff filed a motion for leave to amend her petition and a proposed amendment which would add to her par-

agraph 3 the same allegation contained in the previous,
denied, amendment, and also the allegation that by
using the ultra-sonic machine defendant invaded the field
of the practice of medicine and failed to exercise that
degree of care and skill usually exercised by doctors of
medicine in Council Bluffs. The record shows no objection by defendant to the filing of the amendment.

The court, Judge Cullison, ruled as to the first paragraph of the proposed amendment Judge Everest's order
was the law of the case and such paragraph was disal-
lowed. With reference to the second paragraph of the
amendment the court ruled defendant was under a duty
in the use of the ultra-sonic machine to exercise such care
as a person skilled in such use is required to exercise. No
other ruling was made on plaintiff's motion for leave to
amend. Apparent effect of the ruling was to allow the
second paragraph of the amendment as changed or
amended by the court.

II. The first of two assigned errors is the refusal to
permit the amendment—we understand, the second one.

(3) We think it was error to hold Judge Everest's order
disallowing the first amendment was the law of the case.
As stated, one ground of defendant's resistance to its
allowance is it was not timely. The first ruling may have
been placed upon this ground. Defendant tells us in argument trial of the case was to commence three days after
the first amendment was filed. (this trial was continued
with defendant's consent.) So far as appears, no such
situtation existed when the second amendment was
filed—about 3-1/2 months before trial commenced.
Rubendall v. Brogan Constr. Co., supra, 253 Iowa 652,

657, 113 N.W.2d 265, 268 supports our conclusion on this point.

(4) With reference to the ruling on the second part of the (second) amendment, of course it is true, as defendant argues, the trial court has a good deal of discretion whether to allow an amendment to a pleading after a pleading has been filed responding to it. Rule 88 R.C.P. And the question usually presented on appeal where an amendment has, or has not, been allowed is whether such discretion was abused. We have repeatedly held the allowance of an amendment, especially one like this, is the rule, its denial the exception.

(5) We have also declined to decide whether there was an abuse of discretion in disallowing an amendment where, as here, a law action is reversed and remanded on another ground since, upon the remand, the trial court will have the same discretion to permit an amendment as if the case had not been tried. The presumption is that after the remand such discretion will not be abused. We have so held in a long line of decisions. Webber v. Larimer Hdwe. Co., 234 Iowa 1381, 1389, 15 N.W.2d 286, 290 and citations; Williams v. Stroh Plbg. & Elec., Inc. 250 Iowa 599, 606-607, 94 N.W.2d 750, 755-756, 82 A.L.R.2d 465, 473, and citations; Bashford v. Slater, 250 Iowa 857, 864, 96 N.W.2d 904, 908-909 ("...we may assume the issues will then be clearly resolved, ...").

Our problem is not the usual one, however. The trial court did not disallow the second paragraph of the amendment. He changed it and, as so changed, permitted it to stand. The only apparent basis for the change is that the court felt defendant, in using the ultra-sonic machine, should be held to exercise such care as a person skilled in such use is required to exercise, not the degree of care and skill usually exercised by "M.D.s" in Council Bluffs, as the amendment contemplates. The court may have had in mind, what the evidence shows, that ultra-sonic treatments are frequently administered by nurses, therapists or physicians' aids under the latter's direction and supervision. We are not prepared to hold such common practice would necessarily be illegal or amount to negligence. If this is what the trial court had in mind by changing the language of the amendment little, if any, prejudice could result to plaintiff therefrom.

Defendant tells us the standard of care the trial court announced conforms to our decision in Christensen v. Des Moines Still College, 248 Iowa 810, 817-818, 82 N.W2d 741, 746. There plaintiff recovered in a malpractice action from an osteopathic college for an injury inflicted by a senior student assigned to a licensed practitioner-instructor in the college. In affirming the judgment upon defendant's appeal, the opinon points out the jury was instructed the care necessary was that exercised by senior students of osteopathy at the time and place in question.

Defendant thinks this from the Christensen opinion supports the change the trial court made in plaintff's amendment: "...we may observe in passing that it (instruction) was most favorable to defendant, for the law requires, we think, not only 'the average of the reasonable knowledge, skill and care ordinarily exercised by senior students of osteopathy'...but the exercise of that degree of care, skill and diligence used by the osteopathic profession at that time and place."

We see nothing in the Christensen opinion inconsistent with the claim made in paragraph 2 of plaintiff's amendment.

(6) The general rule is that one sued for malpractice is entitled to have his treatment tested by the rules and principles of the school of medicine in which he belongs, not those of some other school. If he treats the patient with the ordinary skill and care of those of his school he is not answerable for poor results. Wheatley v. Heideman, 251 Iowa 695, 704, 706, 102 N.W.2d 343, 3490350, and citations; Treptau v. Behrens Spa, supra, 247 Wis. 438, 20 N.W.2d 108, 113, and citations; Kelly v. Carroll, 36 Wash.2d 482, 219 P.2d 79, 19 A.L.R.2d 1174, 1182-1183, and Anno. 1188-1198, Anno. 78 A.L.R. 697, 698. See also Anno. 85 A.L.R.2d, 1022, 1023.

(7) But this rule is not applicable here. Plaintiff does not charge defendant with malpractice in treating her back ailment by "adjustment by hand" or "other incidental adjustments." Her complaint is defendant was negligent when he went outside the practice of chiropractic and entered the field of the practice of medicine by administering ultra-sonic treatments. In doing so—and it is admitted he treated plaintiff with an ultra-sonic unit—he is held to the care and skill usually exercised by medical doctors. Treptau v. Behrens Spa, supra; Kelly v. Carroll, supra, and Anno. 19 A.L.R.2d 1188, 1203. See also Anno. 85 A.L.R.2d 1022, 1029.

We think paragraph 2 of the amendment, as tendered, should have been allowed. It is a good allegation of negligence. There is ample authority to support it and none to the contrary has been cited. However, we are also of the opinion that under the change the court made therein the case should have been submitted to the jury.

(8) In view of the remand for a new trial we feel we should express our opinion on defendant's contention that his mere violation of Code section 151.1, I.C.A. as alleged in paragraph 1 of plaintiff's amendment, would not be actionable negligence without proof he failed to exercise proper care in treating plaintiff's foot and such failure cause her injury. We think this contention must be upheld. Anno. 19 A.L.R.2d 1188, 1204-1205. See also Anno. 57 A.L.R. 978.

III. There is substantial evidence defendant negligently failed to exercise such care in the use of the ultrasonic machine as one skilled in the use would exercise. Since, as we have held, use of such machine is part of the practice of medicine we may assume that only "M.D.s" or their assistants, who act under their supervision and direction, are so skilled.

(9, 10) In considering the propriety of the directed verdict of course we give the evidence for plaintiff the most favorable construction it will reasonably bear. It is equally well established that generally questions of negligence and proximate cause are for the jury—it is only in exceptional cases they may be decided as matters of law. Rule 344(f), pars. 2 and 10, R.C.P., 58 I.C.A.

We have said there is ample evidence defendant burned plaintiff's foot by his use of the ultra-sonic machine. We have held the fact a plaintiff is severely burned by defendant's use of an X-ray machine in some evidence in itself the treatment was improper. Shockley v. Tucker, 127 Iowa 456, 458, 103 N.W. 360; Rulison v. Victor X-Ray Corp., 207 Iowa 895, 899, 223 N.W. 745, 747; Berg v. Willett, 212 Iowa 1109, 1112, 232 N.W. 821.

To like effect is Hansen v. Isaak, 70 S.D. 529, 19 N.W. 2d 521, 522. For other somewhat similar decisions see Anno. 41 A.L.R.2d 329, 365.

Our Rulison opinion states: "...if the evidence shows that the plaintiff did suffer an X-ray burn, and that this was her only exposure to an X-ray machine, such circumstance is not only admissible as tending to prove improper use of the machine, but it is also a very persuasive one."

The present case is closely analogous to those just cited. But there is quite a little other evidence of defendant's negligence.

(11) The only witness defendant called was Dr. Hansman, a regular practitioner specializing in internal medicine. He examined plaintiff evidently with a view of becoming a witness. He testified in substance that if proper care were used a sprained ankle of a diabetic could be successfully treated with an ultra-sonic machine. This, together with the fact injury resulted here, is some evidence proper care and skill were not used. George v. Shannon, 92 Kan.801, 142 P.967, Ann. Cas. 1916 B, 338, 340-341. See also Berg v. Willett and Hansen v. Isaak, cited last above.

Plaintiff testified that on each of the three occasions defendant treated her foot with this machine it was applied 15 or 20 minutes and then shut off. Dr. Hansman said the maximum time for applicaton of ultra-sonic therapy on a non diabetic would be five minutes and "the use of this machine on a diabetic for 15 or 20 minutes would be excessive." There is much evidence that feet of a diabetic are more susceptible to burns than are feet of one without the disease, and greater care is required in treating a diabetic with ultra-sonic equipment than is necessary with a normal paitent.

A registered physical therapist—director of a therapy center in Council Bluffs—testifed the duration of an ultra-sonic treatment and the intensity of the heat to be used "should be" prescribed by a medical doctor. Plaintiff's "M.D.," the physical therapist at Mercy Hospital in Council Bluffs, and defendant's expert Dr. Hansman each testified in substance that ultra-sonic treatments were administered, if not by an M.D., only on his prescription as to duration and intensity of the heat to be applied. The hospital therapist said, "We use the machine usually from three to not over ten minutes."

After Dr. Hansman testified as just indicated, there is this record: "Q. Would you say the use of a doctor's prescription is the general accepted use of an ultra-sonic machine in your profession in this community? A. I think that's true.

"Defendant's counsel: That is objected to as irrelevant and immaterial to any issue.

"The court: Sustained."

(12,13) No motion was made to strike or exclude the quoted answer. The objection was not made until after the answer was in and no reason was given for the delay. The ruling did not have the effect of striking the testimony. It remained in the record and is to be considered. Hamdorf v. Corrie, 251 Iowa 896, 903, 101 N.W.2d, 836, 840; Ducummon v. Johnson, 242 Iowa 488, 496, 47 N.W.2d 231, 236; Livingstone v. Dole, 184 Iowa 1340, 1343, 167 N.W. 639. We may add we are unable to agree the question (on cross-examination) was objectionable under the issue raised by the second paragraph of plaintiff's amendment as changed by the trial court. Defendant tells us in argument the true issue is whether he departed from the standard of those qualified to prescribe and apply ultra-sonic therapy. It is not claimed defendant used this machine on plaintiff pursuant to physician's prescription.

Defendant told plaintiff on October 5 he knew nothing about the machine and was just trying it out. We think it may be presumed he had not been trained in the use of such a device. The school of chiropractic he attended would hardly train students to do something outside the field of chiropractic. Dr. Hansman testified in effect that much care is required in the use of such a machine on bony prominences like the ankle and on an older person, as well as a diabetic.

(14) There is other evidence which strengthens plaintiff's claim defendant failed to exercise such care as one skilled in the use of such a machine would exercise. It need not be referred to. We feel enough has been summarized to indicate a jury question was raised.

(15,16) IV. The jury could find the proximate cause of plaintiff's injury was defendant's failure to exercise such care as one skilled in the use of an ultra-sonic machine would use. As stated twice, there is ample evidence the burns on plaintiff's foot were caused by defendant's use of the machine. We think we have pointed out substantial evidence he was negligent in using it. The observation we have frequently made applies here—the issue of proximate cause is ordinarily for the jury where there is substantial evidence of a defendant's negligence. Wilson v. Corbin, 241 Iowa 593, 604, 41 N.W.2d 702, 708, and citations; Daiker v. Martin, 250 Iowa 75, 84, 91 N.W.2d

747, 752. See also cases cited in Anno. 19 A.L.R. 2d 1188, 1194-1196.

Reversed and remanded.

All Justices concur except PETERSON, J., who takes no part.

This is what is meant by chiropractic based on a definition and scope of practice legally sound.

And yet, read this quote from ACA: "Who is the Doctor of Chiropractic?"

"He is a practitioner in a specialized field of healing, trained by four years or more of intensive professional college education to diagnose and treat people. He does not use or prescribe drugs. The form of medicine which he practices is defined technically as "physical medicine."

And read on: "In chiropractic, such folk-lore centers around the miracle performed by the 'founder' of chiropractic, D. D. Palmer, a non-medical man, in helping a poor janitor regain his hearing. This man had lost approximately 90% of his hearing and this condition had prevailed for twenty years. Finding a lump on the backbone, Palmer "adjusted" the area by hand and the patient's hearing was restored. That was in 1895, seventy years ago. So, fork-lore is established."

Read the history stated by D. D. Palmer.

And one more quote will serve to suffice to show the extreme danger. When chiropractors fail to recognize and practice within their own field. "Today's Doctor of Chiropractic", page 7: "The approach in his schooling, the major content of his course of study, and the training he receives in the teaching clinic or hospital attached to his college are geared to diagnosing the patient as a whole person." "The role of the doctor of chiropractic as a general practitioner is large. and growing."

Here is the extreme danger for the chiropractic profession as witness the States of Tennessee and Texas as they eliminated naturopathy because they treated the whole man instead of staying in their rightful field. Naturopathy per se was not eliminated but a medical license is necessary to practice naturopathy.

Study carefully the court decisions on Texas.

Exhibit IV
HENRY SCHLICHTING, JR., Appellant,
v.
TEXAS STATE BOARD OF MEDICAL EXAMINERS,
Appellee
No. A-6617
(Supreme Court of Texas. Feb. 19, 1958)
(Rehearing Denied March 26, 1958)

"Suit by state board of medical examiners to enjoin practicing naturopath from practicing medicine without proper license. The District Court, Midland County, granted temporary injunction and naturopath appealed. The Supreme Court, Garwood, J., held that injunction which was issued after statute recognizing and regulating practice of naturopathy had been declared unconstitutional did not discriminate against naturopath in violation of his state or federal constitutional rights in that naturopath had a recognized healing skill or profession which he was denied the right to practice for lack of a license or any way to procure a license inasmuch as naturopath by meeting requirements for license for practice of medicine could secure such license which in turn would permit him to practice his own peculiar method of diagnosis and treatment.

Affirmed.

1. Statutes - 109

The object of requiring captions on bills is to permit reader of a bill to inform himself of its subject matter without having to read body of bill, this purpose is not accomplished, if caption, for lack of sufficient provision therein or by misleading character of its provisions, does not convey to reader the necessary information. Vernon's Ann. St. Const. art., 3, 5.

2. Statutes - 109.11

Where subject matter of actual amendment is germane to that of provision amended, caption of amendatory bill referring to provision being amended by number only is adequate. Vernon's Ann. St. Const. art 3, 35.

3. Statutes - 109.11

In determining whether amendatory provision having caption referring only to original provision by number was germane to original provision and, therefore, valid, the test is the closeness of relationship of new provisions or substantial changes to what went before. Vernon's Ann. St. Const. art. 3, 35.

4. Statutes - 114 (7)

Amendatory bill giving state board of medical examiners the right to institute an action in its own name to enjoin unlawful practice of medicine at any time was germane to original provision which required state to institute the suit and only after offender was convicted of unlawful practice of medicine, and caption of amendatory bill which contained only general reference to number of original provision being amended was sufficient to satisfy constitutional requirement that subject matter must be included in caption of bill, and amendatory bill was valid. Vernon's Ann. Civ. St. arts. 1434a, 1, 2, 4509; Vernon's Ann. St. Const. art. 3, 35.

5. Injunction - 109

The words "of this act" as used in amendatory act giving state board of medical examiners power to regulate practice of medicine and to institute actions in its own name to enjoin violation of any provisions of the act were intended to mean the entire so called Medical Practice Act, and defendant could not defend suit by state board of medical examiners to enjoin defendant's unlawful practice of medicine without proper license, on ground that amendatory act gave state board authority only as to holders of licenses to practice medicine. Vernon's Ann. Civ. St. arts. 4498, 4509, 4510.

6. Statutes - 230

When a new section has been introduced into a law, it must be construed in view of original statute as it stands after amendment is introduced, and new section and all sections of old law must be regarded as a harmonious whole, all sections mutually acting upon each other.

7. Constitutional Law - 275 (1)
Physicians And Surgeons - 2

Injunction enjoining practicing naturopath from practicing medicine without a license after statute regulating and recognizing practice of naturopathy had been declared unconstitutional did not discriminate against naturopath in violation of his state or federal constitutional rights in that naturopath had a recognized healing skill or profession which he was denied the right to practice for lack of a license or any way to procure a license inasmuch as naturopath by meeting requirements for license for practice of medicine could secure such license which in turn would permit him to practice his own peculiar method of diagnosis and treatment. Vernon's Ann. Civ. St. arts, 4509, 4510, 4590d; Vernon's Ann. St. Const. art. 16   31:U.S.C.A Const. Amend. 14.

McCarthy, Rose, & Haynes, Amarillo, for appellant. Will Wilson, Atty. Gen., Cecil C. Rotsch, John Reeves, Joe R. Carroll, Asst. Attys. Gen., Joseph H. Mims, Dist. Atty., Midland County, Midland, Leonard Howell, County Atty., Midland County, Midland for appellee.

GARWOOD, Justice.

This is a direct appeal pursuant to article 1738a, Vernon's Tex. Civ. Stats., and Rule 499-a, Texas Rules of Civ. Proc., from the District Court of Midland County, by the appellant-defendant, Schlichting, a practicing naturoapth or natureopath, to review, on constitutional and other grounds, temporary injunction granted at the suit of the appellee-plaintiff Texas State Board of Medical Examiners, acting under Art. 4509, Vernon's Tex. Civ. Stats. as amended in 1953, and, in substance restraining the appellant-defendant from practicing the art of healing or treating persons for physical ills.

1. "Art. 4509. The Texas State Board of Medical Examiners shall have the power to appoint committees from its own membership and to make such rules and

regulations not inconsistent with this law as may be necessary for the performance of its duties, the regulation of the practice of medicine, and the enforcement of this Act. The duties of any such committees appointed from the Texas State Board of Medical Examiners membership shall be to consider such matters pertaining to the enforcement of this Act and the regulations promulgated in accordance therewith as shall be referred to such committees, and they shall make recommendations to the Texas State Board of Medical Examiners with respect thereto. The Texas State Board of Medical Examiners shall have the power, and may delegate the said Power to any committee, to issue subpoenas, and subpoenas duces tecum to compel the attendance of witnesses, the productions of books, records and documents, to administer oaths and take testimony concerning all matters within its jurisdiction. The Texas State Board of Medical Examiners shall not be bound by strict rules of evidence or procedure, in the conduct of its proceedings, but the determination shall be founded on sufficient legal evidence to sustain it. The Texas State Board of Medical Examiners shall have the right to institute an action in its own name to enjoin the violation of any of the provisions of this Act. Said action for an injunction shall be in additioin to any other action, proceeding, or remedy authorized by law. The Texas State Board of Medical Examiners shall be represented by the Attorney General and/or the County or District Attorneys of this State. Before entering any order cancelling or suspending a license to practice medicine, the Board shall hold a hearing in accordance with the procedure set out in Article 4506, Revised Civil Statutes of Texas, 1925, as amended by this Act. As amended Acts 1953, 53rd Leg., p. 1029, ch. 426, § 9."

For the reasons more fully appearing below, we have concluded that the injunction in question must be upheld.

The general ground for the injunction is that the appellant-defendant is practicing medicine as defined in Art. 4510, Vernon's Tex. Civ. Stats.,[2] and is doing so without possessing (and thus without having registered with the District Clerk) "the certificate evidencing his right to practice medicine" required by Art. 4498.[3] The restraints of the decree are, of course, conditioned

2. "Art. 4510. Any person shall be regarded as practicing medicine within the meaning of this law: "(1) Who shall publicly profess to be a physician or surgeon and shall treat, or offer to treat, any disease or disorder, mental or physical, or any physical deformity or injury, by any system or method, or to effect cures thereof; (2) or who shall treat or offer to treat any disease or disorder, mental or physical or any physical deformity or injury by any system or method and to effect cures thereof and charge therefor, directly or indirectly money or other compensatons; provided, however, that the provisions of this ARticle shall be construed with an in view of Article 740, Penal Code of Texas, and Article 4504, Revised Civil Statutes of Texas as contained in this Act. Acts 1907, p. 224; Acts 1949, 51st Leg., p. 160, ch. 94, § 21 (b)."

3. "Art. 4498. It shall be unlawful for any one to practice medicine, in any of its branches, upon human beings within the limits of this State who has not registered in the District Clerk's office of every County in which he may reside, and in each and every County in which he may maintain an office or may designate a place for meeting, advising with, treating in any manner, or prescribing for patients, the certificate evidencing his right to practice medicine, as issued to him by the Texas State Board of Medical Examiners, together with his age, post office address, place of birth, name of medical college from which he graduated, and date of graduation, subscribed and verified by oath, when, if willfully false, shall subject the affiant to conviction and punishment for false swearing, as provided by law. The fact of such oath and record shall be endorsed by the District Clerk upon the certificate. The holder of every such certificate must have the same recorded upon each change of residence to another County, as well as in each and every County in which he may maintain an office, or in which he may designate a place for meeting, advising with, treating in any manner or prescribing for patients; and the absence of such record in any place where such record is hereby required shall be prima facie evidence of the want of possession of such certificate. Acts 1923, p. 292; Acts 1931, 42nd Leg., p. 74, ch. 49, § 2."

upon the absence of such license and registration. The appellant-defendant did, indeed, prior to this suit, have a license to practice naturopathy under a statute known as

Article 4590d, Vernon's Tex. Civ. Stats., which purported to recognize and regulate the practice of naturopathy, defining it as " that philosophy and system of the healing art embracing prevention, diagnosis, and treatment of human ills and functions by the use of several properties of air, light, heat, cold, water, manipulation with the use of such substances, nutritional as are naturally found in and required by the body, excluding drugs, surgery, X-ray and radium therapy, and the use of X-ray equipment. However, in Wilson v. State Board of Naturopathic Examiners, 2 ex. Civ.App. 1957, 298 S.W.2d 946, the Austin Court of Civil Appeals rendered judgment declaring that statute to be unconstitutional, from which an application for writ of error was by us refused. Although our action was with notation "no reversible error", we necessarily approved the judgment declaring the statute to be void; and accordingly, since some little time prior to this suit, appellant-defendant has been actually practicing a healing art without a license of any kind.

The facts as above stated are admittedly to be taken as true from the pleadings and affidavits, which constitute the entire record so far as factual matters are concerned. About the only other material fact thus reflected is that the appellant-defendant had not, prior to this suit, been convicted in a criminal proceeding of violation of the laws regulating the practice of medicine. Other than as indicated by the above quotation from Art. 4590d, supra, the record is silent as to the character of naturopathy, its merits or demerits as a method of healing, its difference from other methods, and the character and amount of education and training required for one to become whatever may be meant by the term paracticing naturopath.

The first attack of the appellant-defendant on the injunction is based on the alleged unconstitutionality of the particular provisions of Art. 4509, supra, under which this suit was brought and provisions being additions to and other changes in, the original article made by the amendment thereto known as H.B. 254, Ch. 426, Acts 1953, p. 1029, et seq. The original or unamended article, as it appears in the Revised Statutes of 1925, is also copied in the footnote 4 for purposes of comparison

4. "Art. 4509. Injunction. The actual practice of medicine in violation of the provisions of this title, or in violation of any provision of Title 12, chapter 6, of the Penal Code, shall be enjoined at the suit of the State, but such suit for injunction shall not be entertained in advance of the previous final conviction of the party sought to be enjoined of the violation of any provision of said chapter of the Penal Code. In such suits for injuction, it shall not be necessary to show that any person is personally injured by the acts complained of. Any person who may be or about to be so unlawfully practicing medicine in this State, may be made a party defendant in said suit. The Attorney General, the district attorney of the district in which the defendant resides, the county attorney of the county in which the defendant resides, or any of them, shall have the authority, and it shall be their duty, and the duty of each of them, to represent the State in such suits. No injunction, either temporary or permanent, shall be granted by any court, until after a hearing on complaint is had by a court of competent jurisdiction on its merits. In such suit no injunction or restraining

order shall be issued until final trial and final judgment on the merits of the suit. If on the final trial it be shown that the defendant in such suit has been unlawfully practicing medicine, or is about to practice medicine unlawfully, the court shall by judgment perpetually enjoin the defendant from practicing or continuing the practice of medicine in violation of law as complained of in said suit. Disobedience of said injunction shall subject the defendant to the penalties provided by law for the violation of an injunction. The procedure in such cases shall be the same as in any other injunction suit as nearly as may be. The remedy by injunction given hereby shall be in addition to criminal prosecution. Such causes shall be advanced for trial on the docket of the trial court, and shall be advanced and tried in the appellate courts in the same manner and under the same laws and regulations as other suits for injunction. Acts 1923, p. 291."

the amended version copied as footnote 1. The former, entitled "injunction", deals almost exclusively with injunctions against "the actual practice of medicine in violation of the provisions of this title, or ...of Title 12, chapter 6, of the Penal Code", and provides that such injunction shall be "at the suit of the State". The words "this title" refer to Title 71 dealing with public health, including Chapter 6, Arts. 4495-4512, entitled "Medicine". Admittedly, under this original Article 4509, a suit such as the present could only be maintained by the State, and thus not by the appellee-plaintiff Board, and, moreover, could "not be entertained in advance of the previous final conviction of the party sought to be enjoined". The latter provision also, were it presently applicable, would operate to defeat this suit, there having been "no previous final conviction" of the appellant-defendant. However, the mentioned amendment eliminated this "conviction" provision and also expressly authorized the Board to maintain whatever suits are authorized by the article. The purpose of the constitutional attack on the amendment is accordingly to make this suit subject to the restrictive provisions of the original article, which would prevent its being maintained.

(2) The amendment deals with various articles regulating the practice of medicine and is said to be invalid insofar as Art. 4509 is concerned by reason of the inadequacy of the caption of the corresponding act or bill, which is fully quoted in the footnote. It is said not to "express" sufficiently the "subject" of the amendment in respect of Art. 4509, as required by Art. III, Sec. 35 of the Texas Constitution, Vernon's Ann. St. The object of requiring captions is, of course, to permit the reader of a bill, be he legislator, lawyer, or "man in the street", to inform himself of its subject matter without having to read the body of the bill. Obviously this purpose is not accomplished, if the caption, for lack of sufficient provision therein or by the misleading character of its provisions, does not convey to the reader the necessary information. But, with particular reference to the instant case, it is equally plain that the object of the requirement will not be well accomplished by a caption so detailed as to require anywhere nearly as much time to read as would the body of the act itself.

5. "An Act amending Article 4498a, Article 4499, Article 4499a, Article 4500, Article 4501, Article 4502, Article 4506, Article 4509 and Article 4510 of the Revised Civil Statutes of Texas; providing for repeal of Article 4507 and Article 4508 of the Revised Civil Statutes of Texas; amending Article 741 and Article 743 of the Penal Code of Texas; requiring registration of licensed physicians, providing for duplicate licenses and endorsements, providing for temporary permits, making provision for the compensation of Board members, providing a fee for license and reciprocal agreements, providing fees for examination and provision for revocation, cancellation and suspension, providing for the powers and duties of the Texas State Board of Medical Examiners, repealing all laws and parts of laws in conflict herewith, providing severability; and declaring an emergency." (Emphasis supplied.)

(2) In the instant case, the caption states "amending—Article 4509—." It has been held that such a reference, although not specifying the nature of the amendments, is adequate, where the subject matter of the actual amendments is "germane" to that of the provision amended—the theory being that the reader of the bill will get enough information by looking at the earlier law and the caption of the amendatory bill. Whatever the justification for such a rule, it undoubtedly exists. See Board of Water Engineers of State v. City of San Antonio, Tex. 283 S.W.2d 722, and cases discussed therein.

The difficulty, of course, comes in determining whether the content of the amendment is "germane" to the content of the original act, or portion thereof, in question. "Germane" means, according to a reliable dictionary, "closely allied; appropriate; relevant"; which meaning, in turn, repels that of identity. There is no point in speaking of an amendatory provision being germane unless we mean "different from" as well as "closely allied to" the original provision. Clearly, the relationship that constitutes the germaneness may be of a somewhat general character.

In the Board of Water Engineers case, supra, we held that an amendatory provision prohibiting the withdrawal of water from the Guadalupe or Comal rivers to points outside their respective watersheds was not germane to an original law (Art. 1434a, Vernon's Tex. Civ. Stats.) providing for the organization and corporate powers of corporations "for the purpose of furnishing a water supply...to towns, cities, private corporations, individuals". That statute, as suggested by its number, was what might be termed a "corporation statute", as distinguished from a "water statute"; and, as stated in the opinion, it nowhere used "a word such as 'river', 'stream', 'watercourse', 'watershed', 'dam', or 'lake'." Its subject was remote from the regulation of water rights. Moreover, the caption in question described itself as "amending Sections 1 and 2" of the earlier law, the former section being a general authorization for the kind of corporations above mentioned and containing provisions concerning dividends, sinking funds and the like as being properly includable in the charter, while Section 2 provided for general corporate powers such as that to contract with federal agencies and borrow money. The particular provision of the amending act repeated Section 1 word for word and then added a Section 1a with the provision in question concerning the two rivers. We think the decision is hardly persuasive in the instant case (although it undoubtedly is "germane" to the latter).

(3, 4) It is true that the body of the amendment to Art. 4509 added several provisions about the powers and functions of the Board, which considerably broaden the more or less exclusive subject of the original, to wit, that of abating violations of the laws regulating the practice of medicine by injunction. But this is not to say that the new provisions or changes concerning the original subject of injunctions thus became nongermane to the latter. Even a layman reading the caption of the amendment and the original article, and being interested in the matter of such injunctions generally, should realize that he would quite possibly find something new on the topic by reading the body of the amendment. As above stated, the judicial rule under discussion cannot possibly mean that the amendment, to be valid, must contain nothing new and no change that is important. The test is the closeness of the relationship of those new provisions or substantial changes to what went before. Certainly both of those here in question are closely related to the general subject of the original article. They are also intimately related to—although making vital changes in—the subsidiary or more particular subjects of the old article, to wit, (a) by whom the suit is to be brought and (b) conditions precedent to the suit. A provision that suit may be brought by the appellee-plaintiff Board is closely related to that of the original article requiring it to be brought by the State itself. Both are part of the larger idea of who shall bring the suit, the latter being a subject of both versions. And the deletion by the amendment of the condition precedent of prior conviction is part of the common subject of conditions precedent to the suit. That mere fact that the reader of the amendment caption and old Art. 4509 would not, in reading them, be also reading the changes themselves, is not important. We did not, in the Board of Water Engineers case, supra, mean to imply the judicial rule in question to require that, for the caption of the amending act to be adequate, the reader should be able, by merely referring to the old statute, to tell exactly what changes were being made in it by the body of the amending act.

The cited decision in Texas-Louisiana Power Co. v. City of Farmersville, Tex., Com. App., 67 S.W.2d 235, is not persuasive, since there the express reference in the caption to be a particular in which the named statute was being amended was in effect a misleading statement that this one change was the only one made, a condition not present in the instant case.

We thus conclude that the general reference in the caption to Art. 4509 as being amended is of itself sufficient to satisfy the constitutional requirement. Accordingly, as to the possibly additional reason to uphold the caption, based on the remaining relevant language therein "providing for the powers and duties of the Texas State Board of Medical Examiners", we need make only the following comment: that the quoted clause does not in anywise mislead the reader as to the contents of the body of the act, so as to make this situation parallel to that in the Texas-Louisiana Power Co. case last above discussed.

(5) The next attack on the injunction assumes Art. 4509 to be valid as amended but contends it still not to

authorize prosecution of this suit, since the relevant portion of the article gives the Board merely "the right to institute an action in its own name to enjoin the violation of any of the provisions of this Act" (emphasis supplied) as distinguished from the provision of the original article that "The actual practice of medicine in violation of the provision of this title,....shall be enjoined at the suit of the State..." (Emphasis applied.) The thesis is that, although the original words "this title" may no doubt have been taken to include Arts. 4498, 4509 and 4510, supra, and might thus have forbidden the appellant-defendant doing what he has been enjoined from doing, nevertheless, the words "of this Act" in the amending act cause the amended article to permit injunctions only as to conduct with which the amending act itself deals; and that the conduct so dealt with is only that of holders of licenses to practice medicine, of whom the appellant-defendant admittedly is not one.

(6) Without pausing to test the premise that the particular provisions of the amending act purport to apply only to holders of licenses to practice medicine, we hold that the words "this Act" do not have merely the narrow scope for which the appellant-defendant contends. The argument might have more weight had the act in question not been, as it was, an almost exclusively amendatory measure, plainly designed to change particular articles of, and to fit in with the existing arrangement of, chapter 6 of title 71 more or less as originally enacted by the so-called Medical Practice Act, Acts 38th Leg., Chap. 138 (1923). But, as it is, we think the context in which the words "this Act" occur in the amendment amply justifies the view that what was meant was the Medical Practice

Act as thus amended. We fail to see, as the appellant-defendant sees, something essentially extraordinary in the idea of the Board being the plaintiff in suits against persons such as himself, as distinguished from those who have or have had a license to practice medicine. For example, the State Bar and its appropriate committees, who are expressly authorized by law to proceed in the courts against the practice of law by unauthorized persons, are actually agencies with a peculiar interest in, and thus a special competence for, the exercise of that function, in addition to their functions concerning unethical conduct of authorized practitioners. Our conclusion is a proper applicaton of the rule stated in Shipley v. Flaydada Independent School Dist., Tex. Com. App., 250 S.W. 159, 160, to the effect that:

> "...When a new section has been introduced into a law, it must be construed in view of the original statute as it stands after the amendment is introduced, and it and all the sections of the old law must be regarded as a harmonious whole, all sections mutually acting upon each other."

See also American Surety Co. of New York v. Axtell Co., 120 Tex. 166, 36 S.W.2d 715.

(7) The final contentions of the appellant-defendant are that the injunction violates Art. XVI, Sec. 31 of the State Constitution and the 14th Amendment to the Constitution of the United States. The theory of both contentions is essentially that of discrimination against the appellant-defendant in that he has a recognized healing skill or profession, which he is denied the right to practice for lack of license or any way to procure a license.

The answer to this is the same one made to a complaining masseur by our Court of Criminal Appeals in Germany v. State, 62 Tex. Cr. R. 276, 137 S.W. 130, to wit, that by meeting the requirements for a license for the practice of medicine (as defined in Art. 4510, supra) he could readily procure the latter license, which in turn would permit him to practice his own peculiar method of diagnosis and treatment, there being no law prohibiting a licensed physician so to do. Indeed, the appellant, far from adducing proof that such a course would be an unfair burden on him by reason of the simplicity or other special characteristics of naturopathy, as compared to what is generally understood as the practice of ''medicine'' forthrightly admits that an express requirement conditioning all healing practices on the education and training now required for regular medical practitioners would be valid. The fact that the Medical Practice Act. supra, (see Arts. 4510 and 4504) expressly excepts from its requirements practitioners in fields such as dentistry, chiropractic and chiropody, which occupations are licensed under separate provisions with less burdensome conditions, is mentioned by the appellant but not clearly urged as a factor of unfair discrimination. Certainly there is no evidence in the record, not any judicial knowledge on our part, whereby we might adjudge it unfair or arbitrary to allow, for example, a chiropodist, to get a license upon the less onerous conditions presently required of him and yet require a naturopath to fulfill the more burdensome requirements for the practice of ''medicine''. In this behalf we can only say that from the very words of former Art. 4590d, supra, which appellant cites as an official recognition of naturopathy as a respectable profession, there is an obvious distinction between its field of operations and those of the recognized special or limited professions or occupations aforementioned.

6. "The Legislature may pass laws prescribing the qualifications of practitioners of medicine in this State, and to punish persons for malpractice, but no preference shall ever be given by law to any schools of medicine."

The latter are respectively limited to diagnosis and treatment with respect to rather narrow portions of the human anatomy, while the only limitations in the practice of naturopathy are limitations merely of methods employed. Evidently naturopaths purport to diagnose and treat human ills of all kinds, however limited their methods. In this connection, it was held in the Wilson case, supra, on the strength of decisions of the Court of Criminal Appeals therein cited, that, assuming Naturopathy to be a recognized "school of medicine", to allow it to be licensed upon easier terms than those required for the practice of "medicine", would violate the very provision of the state Constitution under which the appellant now claims relief. The same would be true should we permit it to be practiced without any license at all, while enforcing a statute that requires practitioners of "medicine" to be licensed and on quite onerous conditions. We are cited to no decisions indicating the constitutional provisions in question to be violated by the injunction and hold that they are not.

The judgment of the trial court is affirmed.

The Scope Of Chiropractic Practice
A Legally Defensible Position

It is often heard within the chiropractic profession that if only there were unity all problems would vanish, or at least become greatly diminsihed.

Further, it is submitted that if the ACA and the ICA cannot unite first and then work out a mutually acceptable scope of practice, why then cannot some acceptable statement of scope be worked out between the two groups, and used as a basis of unity?

Should any such eventuality come about, it should be noted that such a scope can only be interpreted according to what is legally defensible rather than what the individual would like to do in his practice. Words can mean one thing to some persons, and something else to others. There could then result mutual agreement without either side intending to practice what the other considers the words of any such scope to mean. How can such an issue be resolved in order that no such misunderstanding arises? There seems to be but one clear way, and that is by making a sincere effort to determine what is meant by "legally defensible" with respect to the scope of chiropractic practice.

Back in 1938, the now famous Boston case reached the Supreme Court of the state of Iowa. Dr. Boston had been practicing in the city of Davenport and allegedly had used physiotherapy, electrotherapy, colonic irrigations and diet. The Iowa Court held against chiropractor Boston stating that such practices were outside the scope of chiropractic. It enjoined him from using physiotherapy, electrotherapy, colonic irrigation, colon hygiene, ultra-violet rays, infrared rays, radionics machines, traction tables, white lights, cold quartz, ultra-violet light, neuroelectric vitalizer, electric vibrator, galvanic current and sinusoidal current, as well as the use of medicine and surgery and prescribing a certain or specific course of diet.

The Wisconsin Court in the celebrated Grayson case (1958) enjoined a chiropractor from a similar list of adjuncts and modalities as not being part of chiropractic practice.

It is, however, argued that states having so-called broad laws would take a different view. Just how different a view? The state of California in two leading cases, People v. Fowler (1938) and People v. Manglagli (1950), sheds some light on what view can be expected in such states.

In Fowler, the defendant contended that section 7 of the Chiropractic Act permitting him "to use all necessary mechanical, and hygienic and sanitary measures incident to the care of the body", was a definition of chiropractic. The court disagreed stating that this language was simply an addition to chiropractic in the state, and went on to stress that these allowances under the chiropractic law could not be used to invade the medical field.

Under the circumstances, it may be well to look at what happened to naturopathy in the states of Tennessee and Texas. In both states, the naturopaths lost their separate licensure laws. Basically, the reason was because such practice is said to differ from medicine only in method, but purports to treat the whole body. The Texas Court particularly, in the case of Schlichting v. State Board of Medical Examiners, pointed out that in such event persons desiring to practice naturopathy might do so after first acquiring a medical degree and license. The court took pains to point out that such was not true of dentistry, optometry or chiropractic, as they were professions limited to a certain part of the body. These cases, occurring in 1947 (Davis v. Beeler) and 1958 respectively, seem to be a warning to those who would seek to care for the entire body without obtaining a medical degree and license.

Other cases occurring since 1964 in Arkansas (Kuhl v. Arkansas State Board of Chiropracitc Examiners), Iowa (Correll v. Goodfellow) and Pennsylvania (Howe v. Smith) lend support to these prior positions, and lead the researcher to the conclusion that the ''legally defensible'' position for chiropractic, as a separate and distinct healing art, is that one which promotes the practice to be adjustment of the spine without the use of adjuncts, modalities, or other methods.

The preceding court cases are reprinted with the permission of West Publishing Company, St. Paul, Minnesota.